THROUGH the FIRE

HOW PEOPLE WITH MENTAL ILLNESS ARE EMPOWERING EACH OTHER

FREDRICK E. VARS

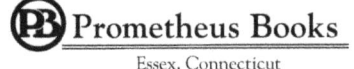

Essex, Connecticut

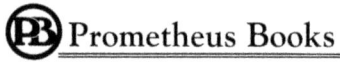

Prometheus Books

An imprint of The Globe Pequot Publishing Group, Inc.
64 South Main Street
Essex, CT 06426
www.globepequot.com

Copyright © 2026 by Fredrick E. Vars

All rights reserved. No part of this book may be reproduced in any form or by any electronic or mechanical means, including information storage and retrieval systems, without written permission from the publisher, except by a reviewer who may quote passages in a review.

British Library Cataloguing in Publication Information available

Library of Congress Cataloging-in-Publication Data available

ISBN 9781493098415 (cloth) | ISBN 9781493087839 (paperback) | ISBN 9781493087846 (epub)

For Kathleen and Kevin

They have been through the fire, and what fire does not destroy, it hardens.

—Oscar Wilde, *The Picture of Dorian Gray*

CONTENTS

Introduction vii

Part I: Illness
CHAPTER 1: Crisis 3
CHAPTER 2: Hospital .18
CHAPTER 3: Jail 34
CHAPTER 4: Outpatient 53

Part II: Recovery
CHAPTER 5: Community 69
CHAPTER 6: Housing .79
CHAPTER 7: Employment 98
CHAPTER 8: Education 116

Part III: Cure
CHAPTER 9: Advocacy 131
CHAPTER 10: Humanity 155
CHAPTER 11: Identity 170

Conclusion 190
Epilogue 197
Acknowledgments 208
Notes 210
Index 239

INTRODUCTION

Mike Autrey was a patient in Bryce Hospital, Alabama's infamous state psychiatric facility, in the 1970s. The staff didn't know how to treat Mike's obsessive-compulsive disorder (OCD), so they sent him to a facility in North Carolina that, Mike was told, had expertise in OCD. It didn't. But it did have one other patient with OCD. Spending time with that patient changed Mike's life: They had similar experiences and could relate to one another. In Mike's view, peer support was the only thing inpatient care was good for.

Mental healthcare in the United States is a disaster. Less than half of people with mental illness receive treatment. Over a million sit in jails and prisons. It is hard enough to live with the symptoms of serious mental illness (SMI).* Society's response to mental illness often makes life even harder. The goal of mental healthcare should be not only to avoid bad outcomes, but also to achieve good ones. The wasted potential of people with mental illness is enormous and largely unrecognized. Nowhere is this more true than within the mental healthcare system.

There is a hidden army of "peers," or people with lived experience of mental illness, helping each other. One study counted 7,467 groups, organizations, and services run by and for people with mental illness or their families. In comparison, there were 4,546 traditional mental health organizations, including hospitals, clinics, and the like. Peer-controlled entities provided services to well over half a million people in 2006. That doesn't even include the many thousands of peers working within the traditional mental healthcare system. In this book I tell some of the

---

* "Serious mental illness" includes primarily schizophrenia, schizoaffective disorder, bipolar disorder, and major depression.

inspiring stories behind these numbers. I also describe key failures in our mental health system that make living with mental illness much harder than it needs to be, and suggest reforms. I propose greater investment in policy interventions that have already been shown to be effective, but my strongest recommendation is for greater peer involvement in policy formation and service delivery.

After his release, Mike Autrey regularly visited Bryce Hospital to provide the same kind of peer support that he received to current patients. The staff at Bryce instructed him not to use the word "recovery" because it gave the patients "false hope." Later, Mike would become director of Alabama's office for mental health peer support, the first of its kind in the country. Mike and the hundreds of "peer specialists" now working in Alabama use the word "recovery" a lot. To Mike, recovery means "creating a life that you want."

Lasting change will require a paradigm shift: recognizing that people with mental illness are people with the same hopes, needs, and desires as anyone else. Mental illness is an illness, not a character flaw. With just a little help through difficult moments, people with mental illness can go on to become effective advocates and mentors for themselves and others. The potential of individuals with mental illness is systematically underestimated and often dismissed altogether. History shows that society simply does not care enough about people with serious mental illness to make meaningful, sustained progress in how they are supported. On many issues and in many settings, we're going to have to help one another. And I do mean "we" literally.

After years of undiagnosed depression and two manic episodes in 2004 and 2006, I finally received a diagnosis of bipolar I disorder. At the time I was working as an associate at a small law firm in Chicago. The stress of a jury trial and an appellate argument contributed to those episodes. Both times the firm waited patiently for me to return to work, but it was clear that a career in litigation would be too triggering in the long term. I worked part-time at the firm while researching and writing an article to present at interviews for law school professor positions (the so-called "job talk"). The firm not only accommodated my disability, but gave me time and space to transition to a new career.

Introduction

The main "hypothetical" case described in my job talk was in fact my own inpatient experience. Technically, during both manic episodes, I "voluntarily" admitted myself into a locked psychiatric unit, even though it was obvious to everyone that I lacked the mental capacity to make that decision. My wife Caroline was with me, but her consent to hospitalization was irrelevant under Illinois law at the time. I argued that that the law should be changed and that there should be a formal mental capacity assessment in that circumstance.

The job talk worked for me. I landed a position teaching law at the University of Alabama, where I have spent my career ever since. I hold an endowed chair and have inspired laws in ten states. I teach and write about mental health law. My best ideas continue to come from personal experience, including the suicide prevention work described at some length in chapter 9. That idea is to empower individuals with a new option to protect themselves against impulsive gun purchase during a suicidal crisis.

Everyone's mental health journey is different. Recovery is not inevitable and is always reversible. When I had two severe mental health crises in my early thirties, I was taken to the hospital and not to jail both times. I had stable housing and employment for nearly twenty years. Then, due to a medication change, I slipped back into crisis and a third hospitalization. I was unable for months to work on this book. I'm lucky to have been able to finish it. In just slightly different circumstances, I could easily have been hospitalized long-term, landed in jail or prison, or become unhoused.

To be clear, this book is not a memoir. Parts of my story appear when discussing topics with which I have had significant direct experience, but the book is grounded on dozens of original interviews of people with diverse experiences living with mental illness. My goals are to destigmatize mental illness, to encourage peer support, and to inspire policy reform. There are stories of remarkable resilience and gutting tragedy, often told by the same person. I have stayed true to the transcripts of our conversations, but I have not independently confirmed the facts relayed in those conversations. And, unless specifically attributed to an interviewee or other source, the suggested policy recommendations are my own.

Stories are the heart of this book, but the recovery model is not just about compassion and maximizing human potential. It is also good economic policy. This book is replete with examples of recovery-oriented policies that save taxpayer money by reducing spending on hospitals, jails, and disability benefits. Many of these policies pay for themselves without even considering the life-changing impact they have on the direct beneficiaries.

Policymakers too often regard the mental healthcare system as consisting of just three levels: crisis, institutionalization, and, for the lucky ones, medical care in the community. But a successful life requires much more than the right meds—it requires things like a supportive community, adequate housing, education, and employment. The chapter order in this book roughly charts a journey through a recovery-oriented mental healthcare system. Genuinely dangerous crises will still sometimes lead to hospitalization or even jail, but many more crises can be de-escalated in the community. Some people cycling through jail or hospital will still need intensive outpatient interventions, but many others can achieve stability outside institutions with housing and community supports. Employment and education are gateways to financial independence and self-esteem. At every stage of recovery, people with mental illness can help one another and themselves through direct service and advocacy in ways that non-peers cannot. Over the long term, we can work to foster recognition of our shared humanity and build a positive identity.

A NOTE ON TERMINOLOGY

The subtitle of this book refers to "people with mental illness." That phrase puts the person first and the condition second. I generally will not use terms like "mentally ill person," any more than I would refer to someone as a "cancerous person." At the same time, I respect any individual's choice to self-identify with a diagnosis-first label. I will often refer to the subjects of this book as "peers" or "people with lived experience." These terms are intentionally vague in order to recognize the validity and value of different types of experiences. Most, but not all, of the "peers" in this book are engaged in direct service or advocacy on behalf of other peers. When that is the case, I generally specify their role with specialized terms like "peer bridger." Some of the people I interviewed for this book reject their formal diagnosis but nonetheless use their interactions with the mental health system to benefit others. "Lived experience" for purposes of this book sometimes includes substance use, homelessness, and other trauma. But the primary focus is on individuals with serious mental illnesses like major depression, bipolar disorder, and schizophrenia. The symptoms of these illnesses, and society's reactions to them, create unique challenges and opportunities. Chapter 1 focuses on one of the most challenging: acute psychosis.

PART I

Illness

CHAPTER 1

CRISIS

"You need to get on the gurney now," the police officer commanded, leaning toward me for emphasis. This may have been the most dangerous moment of my life. I can barely remember it.

* * *

Brandon Marshall was about a decade older than I was when he found himself in a similar situation. Marshall was a forty-three-year-old White man, married, and employed in the tech industry. A neighbor described him as "a really nice guy" who "liked to tinker with motorcycles" and "was definitely into tech." He held a bachelor's degree and a postgraduate degree in computer science. Marshall also happened to be one of a handful of named plaintiffs in a 2011 lawsuit challenging the anti-poaching policies of companies like Apple, Google, Intel, and his former employer, Adobe. The lawsuit alleged that the companies agreed not to call each other's employees to explore hiring, thereby suppressing those employees' job mobility and wages. The case would eventually settle for billions of dollars.

One day in December 2013, Marshall was working for Roku, Inc., a digital media company in Saratoga, California. According to his family, he became "emotionally distressed and disoriented." Before he left the Roku offices, he called his father and asked to be picked up right away. Someone who saw Marshall acting erratically called 911. Fire Department employees encountered Marshall in a parking lot, later describing him as "manic." He agreed to go voluntarily to the hospital. Outside, a paramedic called Marshall's father back to say that his son needed to be taken to the hospital. Marshall's dad said on the phone that he wanted to take his son to the hospital and that he was on his way over.

Before the paramedics or Marshall's father could transport him to the hospital, two uniformed police officers arrived at the scene. They were told that Marshall was a "psychiatric patient." The family claims that even though there was no threat of harm, one officer approached Marshall from behind, which caused him to become "even more upset and agitated." He started fidgeting with his keychain, "a short, thin, rounded aluminum rod." When one of the officers asked him if the keychain was a weapon, Marshall said yes. An officer then charged quickly with gun drawn. Presumably fearing for his life, he swung the keychain at the officers. One police officer shot him in the stomach. Marshall's father heard the gunshot over the phone and heard his son cry out in pain twice before the call ended. He died from the gunshot wound.

Marshall's story is tragically common. According to the police reform organization Campaign Zero, during the four-year period from 2017 through 2020, police killed 356 individuals in the United States where the initial reason for the encounter was mental illness, erratic behavior, or suicide, *and* no weapon or threat to others was noted. It has been estimated that individuals with untreated mental illness are sixteen times more likely than other people to be killed while being approached or stopped by the police.

Police may be afraid of people with mental illness, but those fears are wildly exaggerated: According to the FBI, between 2017 and 2020 only one police officer in the entire country died while "handling [a] person with mental illness." Again, that is the same four-year period in which police killed 356 people with mental illness while responding to mental health calls where no weapon or threat was reported. This massive disparity strongly suggests that police use deadly force against people with mental illness who pose very little risk of killing other people.

These statistics may be surprising. Like the police, the public also overestimates the risk posed by people with mental illness. It is true that people with mental illness have a higher overall rate of violence than the general public. To take an extreme example, people experiencing first-episode psychosis (FEP) have a twenty-fold risk of violence perpetration. The risk is much lower during other phases of illness but remains high for some diagnoses. Schizophrenia is associated with a four to six times greater risk of violence. In other words, some mental illnesses do have a high "relative risk" of violence.

Those correlations between violence risk and mental health status do not necessarily imply causation. Higher levels of violence may be caused by other factors that are also associated with mental illness. For example, people who have a mental illness tend to live in neighborhoods with high concentrations of poverty. There is more violence in those neighborhoods. The landmark MacArthur study followed roughly a thousand people for a year after discharge from psychiatric hospitals. Researchers found a significant independent effect of concentrated poverty on violence, even after controlling for a wide array of individual characteristics. In other words, home address* was part of the explanation for the relatively high risk of violence among people with mental illness.

When the effect of living in a high-poverty neighborhood was combined with the effect of having a substance use disorder, the independent "mental illness effect" disappeared entirely. The former hospital patients who did not also have substance use disorder exhibited the same level of violence as people without a mental illness who lived in the same neighborhood. People with other mental health diagnoses are more likely to have substance use disorder. So, the higher relative rate of violence observed among people with mental illness could be caused entirely by living in violent neighborhoods and being addicted to substances.

Very few studies control for other factors as well as the MacArthur study. Doing so is extremely expensive and, for many purposes, causation doesn't really matter. Erratic behavior is erratic behavior, whether caused by psychosis, alcohol, or illegal drug use. A police officer responding to

---

* Controlling for neighborhood characteristics eliminated entirely a Black–White disparity in levels of violence among people with mental illness. John Monahan, Henry J. Steadman, Eric Silver, Paul S. Appelbaum, Pamela Clark Robbins, Edward P. Mulvey, Loren Roth, Thomas Grisso, and Steven Banks, *Rethinking Risk Assessment: The MacArthur Study of Mental Disorder and Violence* (Oxford University Press, 2001), 58.

a mental health call can see the person, but the officer cannot see the person's medical chart or home address. And a police officer will have already adjusted their risk assessment upward if the interaction is taking place in a high-poverty, high-crime neighborhood. Either way, the decision to use deadly force is based on perceived absolute risk, not an actual diagnosis.

Does the absolute risk of violence during mental health crises justify deadly force? Recall that first-episode psychosis is the most dangerous phase of mental illness. Psychosis is hard to hide, but psychosis alone doesn't justify the use of deadly force. Deadly force is allowed only if "the officer has probable cause to believe that the suspect poses a significant threat of death or serious physical injury to the officer or others." A 2024 article reviewing twenty-two studies of first-episode psychosis found a 13.4 percent prevalence of "any violence." That percentage may be "significant," but the article's definition of "any violence" included conduct that posed no risk of death or serious physical injury, like merely yelling at someone. Only 2.2 percent of violence resulted in "serious injury." A 2 percent chance is not a "significant threat." Deadly force is almost always an overreaction.

* * *

A few months after my release from the hospital, I handwrote an account of my first manic episode. My memory was spotty from the beginning, so I wanted to get some of it on paper before I forgot even more. The story begins the day before I faced off with the police officer. I couldn't find my bike because I was looking in the wrong place. I decided that the bike had been stolen. That thought set in motion a cascade of magical thinking. The missing bike, I believed, "was telling me to slow down, to breathe, to be." For the first time in my life, "it felt as if everything fit, everything had been leading up to this one moment of perfect understanding and bliss." The force of this epiphany knocked me off my feet, literally.

I found myself lying on a sidewalk, laughing and crying. A woman walking a dog stopped to ask whether I was okay. "Yes," I reassured her, "My bike just got stolen—I really loved that bike." "You're mourning your bike—it's important to mourn sometimes," she responded. What the woman said strikes me now as extraordinary, maybe too extraordinary. I know I'm not the most trustworthy source, but I believe that the woman and her dog were real and that something like this conversation actually happened.

There's a reference to "auditory hallucinations" in my medical records from this time, but I'm pretty sure that's a mistake. I don't remember ever "hearing voices" or "seeing things" that other people didn't see or hear. I have a theory about the source of the error in my chart. During mania, I knew God's plan not because I heard Him speak to me in an auditory hallucination, but because I figured it out myself (more on that later). The closest I came to a visual hallucination was mistaking a stranger for one of my former professors, but I was looking down a long hallway without my glasses.

But even if I'm wrong about what the woman with the dog did and said, what's most important is what she didn't do. Notwithstanding my bizarre behavior—I was on the ground sobbing with a ridiculous explanation—she *didn't* call 911. Over the next couple hours, I would interact with many more people as I wandered around my Chicago neighborhood. None of them called 911. If any had, I would have confronted the police outside, alone, manic, and armed with my keys, just like Brandon Marshall experienced.

Instead, after the woman and dog moved on, I picked myself up off the sidewalk. My first idea was to meet my friends across the Midway* at the University of Chicago Law School. I thought that we would search together through the stack of applications from special people, like us, who were qualified to escape the world of suffering and achieve enlightenment. I assumed that my friends had reached nirvana before me. But because I had suffered the longest, my reward would be the greatest: a seat on the United States Supreme Court.

A security guard at the law school asked me whether I was there for the trip to the comedy show. Okay, new plan: We'd all meet at Second

---

* The "Midway Plaisance" is a mile-long stretch of grass connecting two bigger parks on the south side of Chicago. The Midway was the site of the world's first Ferris wheel in 1893. I was on a different kind of ride.

City* instead of the law school. I couldn't sit still on the bus in my manic state, so I got off the bus and climbed into the passenger seat of a nearby car. In the driver's seat was a confused law student. I gave him a hug, then I hopped out of the car and kept moving. My mind locked in on a much better plan, a plan that has saved my life more than once: get back to my wife, Caroline.

The walk from the law school to our apartment should have taken minutes; it took hours. There was so much beauty to absorb on the way. I walked slowly, but the main source of delay was my shifting ideas about *where* to go. The top of a nearby church tower seemed like the perfect place, but the front and side doors were locked. My mind pivoted quickly. I tried the Robie House,† but the door was locked. Eventually, I decided that our apartment had been the ideal place all along. On the way, a person who appeared to be homeless asked me for money. I gave them all the cash in my wallet, about $100, but I kept my ID and credit card.

Finally, I made it back to our apartment, where I expected to find Caroline smiling like Buddha. Instead, she was frantic. Either she hadn't achieved enlightenment yet or she was testing me in some mysterious way. I wasn't sure which, so I decided to hold my cards close to the vest. My mood continued to skyrocket overnight, and by morning I was floridly psychotic and completely out of control. I refused to go to the hospital, so Caroline called our friend Beth for help. Eventually, Caroline had no choice but to call 911. Caroline explained the situation to dispatch and specifically asked for medical assistance. As is typical in these cases, however, an armed police officer was the first to arrive. What could have been a simple medical transport turned into a potentially deadly confrontation.

Today, there is a new national mental health hotline number. Adopted in 2022, the 988 "Lifeline" number is dedicated to suicide and

---

* Second City is a premier venue for improvisational comedy. Notable alumni include Bill Murray, Steve Carell, Jordan Peele, Tina Fey, and Stephen Colbert, among many others.

† The Frederick C. Robie House is an architectural masterpiece designed by Frank Lloyd Wright, which fit well with my delusions of grandeur.

mental health crises (text and chat are also available). The new number is almost certainly saving lives. Overall call volume and answer rate are up significantly as compared to the old, unmemorable 10-digit suicide hotline. The vast majority of crisis center calls are resolved over the phone. Of course, that doesn't include requests for involuntary transport to the emergency department. In most places, those calls are transferred directly to the 911 call center and, by default, trigger a law enforcement response. The 988 number has no impact on cases like mine.

* * *

There is a better way. In some places, when a person in crisis has no weapon and poses no immediate threat, a response team comprised solely of mental health professionals is dispatched. For decades, we have known that this crisis response model is safer for everyone and has better outcomes. The trailblazing Crisis Assistance Helping Out On The Streets (CAHOOTS) program has operated in Eugene and Springfield, Oregon, since 1989. A two-person team consisting of a medic and crisis worker are dispatched in response to mental health calls. Police backup is needed in only a tiny fraction of cases (approximately 2 percent), and no CAHOOTS staff member has ever been seriously injured. This should not be surprising in light of the research, discussed above, finding that there is only a 2.2 percent chance of serious injury during even the most dangerous type of mental health crisis, first-episode psychosis. According to the organization behind CAHOOTS, the program's success depends on the fact that 75 percent of responders have lived experience of incarceration, substance use, neurodivergence, houselessness, and other forms of oppression. Lived experiences like these foster understanding and trust.

Some experts believe that all mental health crisis response teams should be led by peers. In San Francisco, there is a peer on every three-member response team. In addition to having a deeper understanding of mental illness, peers are more likely to live in the same neighborhoods as, and share other demographic characteristics with, the people they serve. Master's degree social workers often live in much different types of neighborhoods than the people they serve. At the same time, it is important to recognize that interactions may be traumatizing for responders with lived experience. Perhaps it's not fair to ask so much of them, but, given the extreme and increasing shortage of mental health professionals, we may not have much choice.

Notwithstanding the well-known success of CAHOOTS, only in recent years have a significant number of jurisdictions begun to implement similar approaches to crisis response. In many areas, there aren't nearly enough specialized teams to meet demand. Recently approved federal funding for programs like this should help, but federal funding is precarious and that money won't be enough without substantial investments at the state and local levels. Ironically, CAHOOTS has saved Oregon millions of taxpayer dollars because the program is less expensive than a police response and much less likely to result in jail or prison. Savings in a single year have been estimated at $8.5 million. Here is a cheap and easy way to reduce killings by police, but few places have adopted it.

It is impossible to identify with certainty any specific individual whose life was saved by a non–law enforcement crisis response. We can never know for sure what would have happened if the police had arrived first. That said, the following true story illustrates how peer-led crisis response can dramatically reduce the chances of an encounter turning deadly. Vania Mendoza, a peer supervisor with San Francisco's crisis response team, told me this story. It begins with a striking juxtaposition: At a street corner atop one of those beautiful hills in San Franciso, a young Black man named Tyler* is yelling loudly at pedestrians and swinging around a large, serrated knife. Someone calls 911. Because Tyler is wielding a knife, dispatch sends law enforcement, *not* a crisis team. The police will arrive just a few minutes later.

But by an almost unbelievable stroke of good luck, Vania's crisis response team happens to be driving on that block at that moment, in between its own assignments. When Tyler, who is a regular client of the team, recognizes their vehicle, he throws down the knife even before the vehicle stops, comes over, and starts venting to the team about his stresses and struggles. They give him some snacks. Vania explains that

---

* Not his real name.

people with mental illnesses can get "hangry," just like everyone else. In about two minutes, he's "de-escalated himself."

Tyler is calm now, but he's not out of the woods just yet. Three police cars with lights blaring arrive nearly simultaneously. An officer explains that they got a call about a knife. Somewhat hilariously, Tyler now feels comfortable enough to start directing the scene, telling the cops that they can leave: "We're good here. I'm fine. There was a problem, but it's not a problem anymore." Understandably, the cops still want the knife. Vania points to the knife a dozen or so feet away, under another vehicle. Now Tyler wants to be helpful, so he starts walking over to the knife to get it for the police. Alarmed, Vania sees what's happening and distracts Tyler by restarting their conversation. The cops retrieve the knife, and the crisis response team gives Tyler a ride back to his neighborhood. It's quite possible that the crisis response team saved Tyler's life once, or maybe twice. Either way, this story illustrates how effective a peer-led, non–law enforcement team can be in defusing a potentially dangerous situation. No injury, no arrest, no hospitalization.

It is important to emphasize that, unlike the police, peer-led crisis response teams do not have the power to make an arrest or to force someone into an ambulance. As we will see in chapter 3, jail is perhaps the worst possible place for a person with a mental illness. Emergency rooms are generally better, but hospitals have their own deep pathologies (chapter 2). Peers can always call for backup if needed. So along with saving lives at the scene, avoiding the criminal justice system and the inpatient mental healthcare system are huge advantages of peer-led crisis response.

Peer-led crisis response teams may not be feasible in low-population-density areas. There may not be enough peers or non-peer providers. Oklahoma pioneered the use of iPads to address this issue. Police officers use the devices to connect individuals in crisis directly to an on-screen mental health therapist. The program has helped reduce adult psychiatric emergency department visits by more than 90 percent. The success of that program led lawmakers to distribute connected iPads to homeless shelters and directly to people with mental illness. Easy access to therapy both prevents crises from developing and defuses crises when they arrive, with no need for in-person crisis response.

Peer-led crisis response saves money as well as lives. This is especially true when places take an integrated approach, including specialized mobile teams and mental health stabilization facilities. The cost savings from collaboration can be breathtaking. In Maricopa County, Arizona, a $100 million investment in crisis care resulted in savings of $260 million in psychiatric inpatient spending and thirty-seven full-time equivalents of police officer time and salary.

* * *

Notwithstanding the positive results of CAHOOTS and programs like it, in most parts of the country today, an armed police officer will still be the first to respond to a call for help during a mental health crisis. This is an incredibly dangerous situation. My wife and I certainly didn't appreciate the magnitude of the risk at that time. And while my survival was not guaranteed, my chances were a lot better than most. Mostly by luck, I had a long list of advantages.

The officer at our door could see immediately that I was unarmed. It's a little embarrassing, but now I feel fortunate that I was compelled by some delusion or another to have taken off all my clothes a few minutes before the cop arrived. I had no keychain, or anything else, in my hands. That fact alone may have been enough to save my life. According to a *Washington Post* database, 84 percent of people shot by the police during a mental health crisis were armed. Without a weapon, I did not pose a "substantial threat" of serious bodily harm, so the officer, if pressed, may have reached for a Taser instead of a gun. That's what happened a few years later when a Chicago police officer used a Taser against an unarmed, naked, sixty-five-year-old woman with bipolar disorder and schizophrenia. That seems like an unjustified use of force, but it's better to be stunned than dead.[*]

---

[*] Tasers are less lethal than firearms, but a significant number of people die after being Tased by police. Katie Conlin, "Shock Tactics: The Taser Cases," Reuters Investigates, accessed June 5, 2025, https://www.reuters.com/investigates/special-report/usa-taser-database/.

My odds of survival were higher for demographic reasons as well. I am White, I was over thirty years old, and I was wealthy enough to be standing in a nice apartment, in a low-poverty neighborhood. Almost exactly ten years after my encounter with law enforcement, a Chicago police officer shot and killed Laquan McDonald. Like me, McDonald had been "behaving erratically." Unlike me, he was only seventeen years old, Black, outside, and in a less advantaged neighborhood. It is true that McDonald was holding a knife, but he was walking away from the police when an officer—who had been on the scene for less than thirty seconds—shot him sixteen times. Most of these shots were fired *after* McDonald had fallen to the ground.

The McDonald case drew intense media attention only a year after the event when a court ordered the police department to release a damning dash-cam video. Officer Jason Van Dyke was charged and convicted of second-degree murder. Van Dyke was sentenced to almost seven years in prison, but he was released after less than half of that time. The case and cover-up prompted a federal investigation of the Chicago Police Department, resulting in a consent decree (a legally binding agreement between consenting parties) to improve transparency and regulate disproportionate police conduct. The department has made progress in some areas but, as of 2024, was still not in compliance with the consent decree. Without the video, there likely would have been no accountability, either for the officer or at the departmental level.

The biggest advantage of all was that, unlike McDonald, I was not alone. My wife Caroline, a doctor, was on my side of the door trying to calm me down and convince me to get dressed. My friend Beth, a lawyer, had arrived at that point and was in the hallway explaining the situation to the police officer. That's right: I had my own personal doctor and lawyer communicating with law enforcement on my behalf. It is hard to imagine circumstances more favorable for surviving a police encounter during a mental health crisis.

Even with this embarrassment of advantages, there was one wild card that could have killed me: the content of my delusions. The overwhelming majority of people experiencing first-episode psychosis are not violent at all—as noted above, an average of 86.6 percent combining twenty-two studies. Still, my delusions conflicted with reality in dangerous ways. It is ironic that the period during which I felt most in control of my life was the period I was least in control. I may not have been seeing or hearing strange things, but I was certainly believing them. A delusion is often defined as a fixed false belief. During mania, my delusions were more real to me than anything else. Other thoughts, beliefs, memories, and even present sense impressions didn't stand a chance. If a delusion contradicted reality, then it was reality that had to give way. The sky was green no matter how blue it looked.

The delusion of being the one in control may seem like a particularly absurd delusion—and it is—but a simple game can illustrate. Have you ever tried to impress the other people in the car by turning a red light green with your mind? There's a trick that always works. It's not stealing a glance at the lights in the opposite direction or memorizing the timing—those are obviously cheating. What works every time is redefining success. You point and say "Now," but the light doesn't change. Just keep pointing and saying "Now" over and over until the light changes. Then, convince yourself that you were intending from the beginning to change the light on the fifth "Now," not the first one. Voilà, you changed the light with your mind! Your kids in the back seat won't fall for it, but you will, if you're delusional in the way I was.

Moving the goalposts in this way was the key move for me to sustain a delusion of control during my manic episode. There was no such thing as a new fact that didn't conform to my plan. There was only the seamless and endless revising of the plan to become ever more beautiful and complete. Or, as I put it in my journal, "I was constantly fitting the puzzle pieces together in different and contradictory ways, adding and subtracting pieces as well." This was not a superpower I wasted on something as trivial as streetlights—no, no, I aimed much higher. In the Bible, Jacob wrestled God all night and eventually prevailed. Never much of a wrestler, I challenged God to a game of poker instead. My version of poker was unique: I would win if I looked at the digital clock at the exact moment it switched over to the next minute. I went all in, wagering what I loved most in the world: my wife Caroline. If I lost, God would take her away from me forever. If I won, God would grant me one wish. Inevitably, I won.

> *What I did in the showdown was what He should have done the first time—I asked for more time. In that extra time I wished for an infinite number of infinitely good universes. This, I thought, was like wishing for more wishes. It maximized goodness. There would be no more pain and suffering. But I guess my wish didn't cover our own universe because it didn't change perceptibly. And I wonder now whether I didn't take this lack of change as a sign that there actually wasn't any room for improvement. Writing now it seems as if God and I did essentially the same thing—we stalled. Although I have no recollection of it, Caroline tells me I was screaming, "This is the best of all possible worlds!" in the hospital later that day. I do remember feeling that way.*

It was only a few moments after the poker game that I opened the door and stood face-to-face with the police officer. The delusion of control is dangerous when it butts up against someone with real power, especially someone armed with a gun and handcuffs. Insisting that you are in charge, and that the police officer is not, is a perilous thing to do. In some circumstances, failing to follow a police command can prompt deadly force even if psychosis alone does not. If just walking away can get you killed, as it did Laquan McDonald, then direct confrontation is a crazy thing to do.

To make matters worse, I knew that I was not just omnipotent, but also omniscient. Cops must love that, too. I understood how and why God had created an imperfect world, hoping it would be perfected with time: "So he created variety and vastness, along with the laws of nature that make evolution possible." I alone could see the full plan. In that moment, I was "smarter than God." I was all-knowing and all-powerful, so why did I obey the command of a mere mortal cop? I had already dismissed urgent pleas by Caroline, Beth, and the EMTs to get on the gurney before the cop told me to. A day or two later, while I was still manic, a nurse on the psych ward told me it was against the rules to take the entire bowl of fresh fruit back to my room. "We both know rules are meant to be broken," I boldly responded. She let me take the bowl rather than pushing back. I don't think the officer would have been that understanding.

In 2021, the *New York Times* examined fatal traffic stops and concluded that in many cases, police responded "with outsize[d] aggression to disrespect or disobedience." Officers even have a name for it: "contempt of cop." Less than two years later, Memphis police pulled over a twenty-nine-year-old Black man named Tyre Nichols. During thirteen minutes of the encounter captured on video, police officers issued seventy-one commands that the *Times* described as "confusing, conflicting and sometimes even impossible to obey." Nichols's failure to comply led to escalating force. Police beat Nichols to death.

Delusions of grandeur are dangerous on their own, but paranoia multiplies the risk. Just a few days after the encounter with the cop, I was wandering the psych ward at night. They usually just let me wander, but I must have been making too much noise that night because someone called security. The guards tried to convince me to get out of the hall and into the TV room. They were probably trying to get the noise level down so the other patients could sleep, but I knew that their real plan was to isolate me, then sodomize me with nightsticks. When I think about this moment, I can still feel the terror. I have only a spotty memory of what happened next. I must have physically resisted because I think I was held face down on a bed and forcibly injected with a sedative.

Days earlier, my delusions felt great. When the officer leaned forward and commanded me to get onto the gurney, I did. I have no idea why I deferred to the officer—after all, I thought I was smarter and stronger than God. If I had perceived the police officer to be a threat, like the hospital security guards just days later, I would have fought back. I wouldn't have been able to stop myself. My delusions were in control, not me.

It is disturbing to realize that you are alive because of outrageously good luck. I had many built-in advantages when I stood face-to-face with the police officer, including age, race, and wealth. But Brandon Marshall too had these. The most critical factor for me may have been timing. No one who observed my bizarre behavior when I was wandering alone in public called 911, so I ended up facing law enforcement later, in our apartment, unambiguously unarmed and flanked by my own personal doctor and lawyer. Even then, survival was not assured. My grandiose delusions still could have gotten me killed—just days later during the same manic episode, I scoffed at one authority figure and physically resisted others in uniforms. As great as he was, I doubt the police officer at our door would have liked either response.

TAKEAWAYS

- Police kill far too many people each year responding to mental health calls.
- These interactions are potentially dangerous, but the absolute risk of serious injury is tiny.
- In most cases, peer-led crisis response teams are better at avoiding injury, death, and needless trips to jails and hospitals.
- As the next two chapters will show, jail and hospital are extremely bad options.

CHAPTER 2

HOSPITAL

Jon Brock was a resident at Alabama's Bryce Hospital in the 1960s. After six rounds of painful shock treatment, Jon convinced his older sister to withdraw consent. When a guard came to collect Jon for another round, he told the guard that consent had been withdrawn. The guard heard Jon but said nothing and took him anyway. Jon told an attendant about the withdrawal of consent and got the same blank look. The attending physician didn't care either. His response was: "Get up on the table." Jon remembers "a slam of the electricity through [his] head."

***

There is no way to understand the current state of inpatient psychiatric care in the United States without understanding history. As was true in the Civil Rights Movement, Alabama played a leading role. The Alabama Insane Hospital was founded in 1859. It was later renamed Bryce Hospital. By the 1870s, virtually every state had at least one comparable state-funded psychiatric hospital. For many years, conditions for residents at Bryce were good, often better than at home or in the community.

Driven by underfunding and overcrowding, however, Bryce deteriorated dramatically during the first half of the twentieth century. The patients themselves sounded the alarm in 1951 in a remarkable weekly newsletter called *The Bryce News: Of the Patients, By the Patients, For the*

Patients. The third issue reported that Alabama spent only $1.29 per patient per day, well below the national average. "Alabama owes it to her mentally ill to bring her appropriation to the nation's average or much nearer than the present." The patients also listed some of the outrageous staffing ratios, including one psychologist for every 2,140 patients. A related criticism was overcrowding. According to the patients, Bryce was the most overcrowded state hospital in the country, with a patient census well over double its rated capacity.

Conditions got even worse during the next twenty years. One journalist described Bryce Hospital as a "hellhole" with human feces on the walls and urine soaking the floors. Photos show patients strapped to rocking chairs. In 1971, Bryce housed approximately five thousand people with only three psychiatrists on staff. Some have said that Bryce in this timeframe resembled a warehouse more than a hospital. While the "warehouse" description accurately captures the lack of meaningful treatment, it misses the reality of affirmative mistreatment, including electroshock therapy and solitary confinement.

When I asked Jon Brock what people don't understand about Bryce in that era, he paused for a moment, then said:

For lack of a better way to say it, the experience of being committed to an insane or a mental hospital, particularly during those times. . . . You were voided. . . . You cannot own property. You cannot buy and sell anything that by default was in truth yours. You could not marry. You could not take any legal action whatsoever on your behalf. Legal actions were things that were done to you. I don't want to say for you, but were done to you. Whatever human capacities you had that were recognized in all settings or in these settings, you're no longer counted as having that capacity. You were legally no longer a person.

In 1970, guardians of patients at Bryce filed a class action lawsuit against the State of Alabama called *Wyatt v. Stickney*. The next year, federal judge Frank Johnson announced for the first time in U.S. history that involuntarily hospitalized psychiatric patients have a constitutional right to treatment: "To deprive any citizen of his or her liberty upon the altruistic theory that the confinement is for humane therapeutic reasons and then fail to provide adequate treatment violates the very fundamentals of due process." The right to treatment was a huge legal victory, but even bigger was the right to have rights.

The state initially agreed to a detailed set of minimum requirements, including 1 psychiatrist for every 125 patients (down from almost 1,700). Almost immediately, however, the state reversed course and fought vigorously against implementing the very changes it had just agreed to make. In the end, it took thirty-three years for Alabama to come into compliance with the so-called "Wyatt standards." The state's primary strategy was not to hire more psychiatrists, but rather to bring down staffing ratios by releasing patients.

This "deinstitutionalization" occurred all over the country, not just in Alabama. Bryce was an extreme case, but most state psychiatric facilities were overcrowded and provided little treatment. Nationwide between 1970 and 2018, the number of beds in state psychiatric hospitals fell by 84 percent. That oft-cited statistic is a bit misleading. In more recent decades, the number of psychiatric beds in general hospitals and beds in private specialty facilities has increased—probably not by enough to make up the difference, but the exact numbers are unknown.

* * *

One product of the inpatient bed shortage in hospitals is longer wait times in emergency departments. Currently, many individuals in acute mental health crises are stuck "boarding" in emergency departments for days, weeks, or even months, until an inpatient bed becomes available. The number of people affected is enormous. For example, in North Carolina on any given day in January 2023, an average of 350 people waited in emergency rooms for psychiatric beds.

Here's how one peer advocate described her experience to me: People were *screaming and yelling, and no doors, and it was horrible, you know, they wouldn't give me my regular medication for my blood pressure. It was a nightmare, and I stayed there for the week of Martin Luther King's Birthday. That, and you know nothing was open. Nothing was being done. I don't even remember what we ate. My kids couldn't find me for three days. They didn't know if their mother was alive or not for three days.*

Being in the emergency department for a prolonged period is never a good option, but it is a particularly bad option for psychiatric patients. The whole design is wrong. "The ER is a bright, loud, noisy, sometimes very chaotic, always changing environment that's on 24/7, 365," explained Dr. Kevin Steinl, head of emergency medicine for one North Carolina healthcare system. Conditions like these exacerbate mental health crises.

Some emergency departments respond to behavioral problems with seclusion and restraint. In a 2018 lawsuit against the state of New Hampshire, a group of "boarded" individuals claimed that many of them were "detained in conditions that are tantamount to solitary confinement." Rather than improving its emergency departments, New Hampshire initially paid lawyers to defend the lawsuit, just as Alabama had done fifty years earlier in the *Wyatt* case.

New Hampshire only agreed to settle the case after hospitals joined the suit and convinced the trial court that the state was unlawfully seizing their property by forcing them to hold the patients. Of course, the hospitals could have added inpatient psychiatry beds, but that would have cut into their profits because each psychiatric hospitalization earns far less than using the bed for surgical or other medical purposes. The financial cost of providing care apparently counted for more than the human cost of not providing it. To its credit, the State of New Hampshire chose not to appeal but instead announced that it would eliminate emergency room boarding within two years as part of a comprehensive plan. In December 2024, the state reported that there were no adults boarding in ERs waiting for inpatient psychiatric care.

Some time in emergency rooms is inevitable, and long waits remain in other states. The number of visits is simply too large. Nationally, emergency departments receive over ten million psychiatric patients each year. There is a proven way to provide much better emergency room care for people during mental health crises. In 2012, Doctor Scott Zeller created the first EmPATH unit, which is short for Emergency Psychiatric Assessment, Treatment, and Healing. Zeller converted a large waiting room into a calm space with soft lighting, TVs, and card tables. Now, arts and crafts are also encouraged. Some healthcare professionals predicted that putting patients in crisis together in a shared space would cause them to agitate one another. The opposite turned out to be true: Behavioral problems became significantly less frequent. EmPATH staff are trained differently as well. They don't try to solve every problem with medication. Sometimes, staff members just ask patients what they need. It could be something as simple as getting an item their family left for them.

Respecting patients' autonomy, even those in crisis, can produce better outcomes. In one research study, Zeller asked mentally ill patients in emergency departments to graph their well-being over time. Things got better and worse, they reported, but the overall trend was in the wrong direction. Nearly every patient described the worst of it as the moment they "lost control." Zeller's response? Give patients back a sense of control. Now, patients in EmPATH units can get themselves water and basic supplies, for example, rather than depending entirely on busy staff. Small movements toward thoughtful patient-centered care can have big impacts.

A key component of the EmPATH model is to reduce the amount of time patients wait to be seen by healthcare professionals. This shift can also result in higher revenues for emergency departments since patients faced with long waits often leave before being assessed. The patients who leave will likely be back, and in worse condition. When patients receive care more quickly and humanely, fewer end up needing hospitalization. One Minneapolis EmPATH unit reduced hospital admissions for mental health crises from 40 percent to 15 percent. Repeat visits also go down with EmPATH units. The most important goal of the model is to "formulate an appropriate disposition and aftercare plan." In other words, don't just kick the can down the road.

Another approach to dealing with mental health crises avoids the hospital entirely. In 1989, New York state authorized stand-alone psychiatric emergency programs. Better late than never, Alabama since 2020 has committed funds to build six 24/7 mental health crisis centers around the state. People can voluntarily come into these centers for services. In addition, first responders can bring people to the centers instead of to jails or emergency departments. At each center, the individual can receive stabilization, evaluation, and psychiatric services. There are beds available for stays up to a week. All the crisis centers in Alabama have peer support specialists on staff.

A pilot study in Utah demonstrates the promise of the crisis center approach. During the first seven months the Utah center was open, it provided services to 228 people. About half of those individuals were dropped off by law enforcement—among those, 45 percent would have gone to jail but for the center. Nearly 20 percent would have gone to the emergency department. Because of the center, people received appropriate treatment more quickly, and healthcare system costs went down.

* * *

Jesse Mangan first interacted with the mental health system at age nineteen. It was the beginning of his sophomore year at the University of Massachusetts Amherst. He had lost a bunch of weight in the previous year, but it had been gradual and he didn't really notice. His goal was not to lose weight, but simply to eat healthy and exercise. Family members began to express concerns. He thought they were just exaggerating the issue—that is, until he started feeling less tolerant of pain, cold all the time, and experienced decreases in energy level and ability to focus, and a compulsion to exercise. Jesse filled out a survey and met all the criteria for an eating disorder. He tried to join a peer support group, but the group didn't allow men.

Jesse's next attempt to get help was an appointment with a nutritionist at student health services. He showed up promptly at 9:00 a.m. on a Wednesday in October 1999. What happened next radically changed the course of his life. The nutritionist called in a doctor. The doctor told Jesse he was in such an extreme condition that he might die if he moved too much. Then the doctor called in a psychologist. Jesse's brother was in the room ready to drive him to whichever hospital they recommended, so it was a shock when EMTs (emergency medical technicians) strapped Jesse to a gurney and drove him away in an ambulance. They deposited Jesse in a locked psychiatric ward and told him he couldn't be released until Monday at the earliest.

Jesse was confused. Why the gurney and ambulance? The psychologist later explained that he didn't trust Jesse's brother to drive him to the hospital because the psychologist had observed the two of them laughing earlier that day. Why the locked psych unit? The psychologist's stated justification was that Jesse was suicidal. The opposite was true: Jesse was afraid of dying and wanted treatment. Later, the psychologist admitted that he didn't actually believe Jesse was suicidal, but that saying so was the easiest way to get him into a facility. Plus, it was 5:00 p.m. and the psychologist had to pick up his child at soccer, or something like that, Jesse recalls.

Things went even farther downhill. Jesse would be involuntarily hospitalized two more times. In the end, he thinks all of this "treatment" did more harm than good. The anorexia symptoms faded after a few years, but he has suffered from post-traumatic stress disorder (PTSD) starting from that first day to the present. For fear of being hospitalized again, Jesse has not seen a doctor for the past fifteen years. Twice, he almost died in his apartment from low blood sugar. The second time he didn't even cry out for his sleeping wife because he thought she might call an ambulance.

***

Bryce Hospital in 1970 did not have the resources to provide adequate inpatient care. There were too few staff and way too many patients. Some patients had no business being hospitalized at all; they weren't even mentally ill. The named plaintiff in the landmark right-to-treatment case was among them. Ricky Wyatt had been sent to Bryce at age fourteen. His only diagnosis was delinquency. This was possible because probate judges at that time were authorized by statute to send any individual that they deemed "sufficiently defective mentally" to facilities like Bryce.

Harry London was another patient at Bryce who didn't belong there. I know nothing else about London, but I cannot believe a "mentally defective" person could have written this poem (which appeared in the third issue of *The Bryce News*):

I WAS MYSELF
I am myself—not yet, but shall be;
Less than I become, more than I do;
Equal to my friends; less than my love;
More than my work, less than my poetry;
Making and unmaking myself—man;
Rebuked and doubted and the between,
And hide myself and give myself away;
And say less than I think, more than I mean.
I built a house which I may not inhabit,
And sow a vineyard which I may not reap,
And ponder with problems which are not my own,
And read a language I may never speak—
And joke and err and plan to be forgiven.
I am all these I do; like many, have
Offenses more than thoughts; but no helpers,
Except the words I cast into the mails.

In 1974, an Alabama federal court examined the question of who could be involuntarily committed and held that merely having a mental illness was not enough. The state also had to prove that the person "poses a real and present threat of substantial harm to himself or to others." And if danger to self but not others is the basis for commitment, the state must also prove that the person lacks the mental capacity to make their own decision regarding hospitalization. Over 1,200 patients were released just a year after this opinion. Every state now requires a showing of dangerousness for involuntary hospitalization—also commonly referred to as "civil commitment." Both the right to treatment and the dangerousness requirement originated from the principle that people don't forfeit their right to liberty just because they have a mental illness. These two judicial decisions were a logical extension of the Civil Rights Movement of the 1960s: Discrimination based on mental disability is like discrimination based on perceived race or gender. In each case, a person is deprived of their rights because of a status they didn't choose.

I have a unique perspective on this history. From the door of my office, I can see the historic Bryce Hospital building. I once took a tour of parts of the hospital that were no longer in use. I noticed an empty wooden coffin leaning against a wall in the crumbling auditorium. "What's that doing here?" I asked. "Yeah, they used to make those themselves," the guide replied. For most of its history, Bryce was truly a place where patients came to die, not to get better. If I had been born sooner, I could well have died as a patient at Bryce. During my first two manic episodes, I spent twenty-eight days of my life in a locked psychiatric ward. I always tell the exact number of days because I experienced each day as a new injury, and I tried every day to get out. I know now that I needed to be confined during those episodes, but the trauma was nonetheless real. Toward the end of my first hospitalization, one doctor-in-training casually said I could be discharged "today, tomorrow, or the next day." I was enraged. It might not have mattered to him which exact day I was released, but it sure as hell mattered to me. Jon Brock observed the same thing when he went back to Bryce to mentor other patients: they all knew exactly how long they'd been there (one for decades), but They had no idea when they'd leave. Jon explained that everyone at Bryce was trying to get out, not to get better.

The cost of providing adequate inpatient care was an important driver of deinstitutionalization, but another important factor is the development of new medications that can stabilize patients faster. More effective treatments mean that psychiatric units are no longer dead ends; now, psychiatric hospitalization is usually just a pit stop. Patients stabilize enough to be released relatively quickly. This has radically changed the nature and duration of involuntary hospitalization. Most stays now last only a few days—no need to make your own coffin. As a result, notwithstanding the massive reduction in public inpatient beds, the number of civil commitments has barely changed. That's only possible because each bed is being used over and over, rather than serving as a final destination for just one person.

It is estimated that approximately 40 percent of individuals discharged from inpatient psychiatric care return within a year. If the goal is to reduce future hospitalizations, civil commitment is not working very well. There are, however, other goals. Civil commitment of a person who presents an immediate danger to self or others reduces the risk of harm in the short term. This would be true even if no treatment were provided: Units are generally locked and do not contain objects commonly used in suicide attempts. Unfortunately, involuntary hospitalization will sometimes be needed, at least until we find and implement other effective ways to defuse dangerous crises.

Civil commitment has long been the default approach to mental health crises in every state, even though it entails a massive deprivation of liberty. The legal and ethical questions raised by that trade-off have been explored in countless books and articles. Many doctors and others assume that involuntary hospitalization benefits patients beyond the acute crisis. There is, however, little evidence of any such benefits.* Still, until we have robust alternatives to manage mental health crises, forced hospitalization may sometimes be inevitable. The "revolving door" phenomenon is not. The key is connecting patients at discharge to resources in the community. Until that regularly happens, involuntary hospitalization amounts to just kicking the can down the road.

Programs that prevent the next crisis are the best way to avoid forced treatment and costly inpatient stays, not to mention the human suffering caused by the crisis itself. One solution employs people who have themselves successfully navigated the system—known as "peer

---

* Alarmingly, one study found that "people who felt they were coerced into being hospitalized against their will were more likely to attempt suicide after being released from the hospital." Peter Simons, "Involuntary Hospitalization Increases Risk of Suicide, Study Finds," *Mad in America*, June 24, 2019, https://www.madinamerica.com/2019/06/involuntary-hospitalization-increases-risk-suicide-study-finds/.

bridgers"—who are uniquely able to assist individuals leaving the hospital. Social workers and other professionals can provide information; peers can also provide deeper understanding through firsthand experience, an ongoing mentoring relationship, and inspiration. Evidence from a long-standing peer bridger program in New York suggests that the program substantially reduces the incidence of rehospitalization, from around 40 percent to 29 percent.

* * *

"Where are you? I'm coming to get you."

Those words saved more than one life. Anna Fiscus-Surita started self-injuring at age ten. Before reaching adulthood, Anna had experienced sexual assault by a family member, substance use, and a suicide attempt. A stay in a psychiatric hospital felt to her like a "punishment," not a path toward healing; "It just reiterated to me that I was broken and I deserved to be treated in certain ways." She previously identified more with substance use and criminal justice involvement, but has come to recognize her deep-rooted trauma and complex PTSD. At age eighteen, Anna began cycling through jail, hospitals, and the street as a result of her substance use and other mental health problems.

That vicious cycle continued for nearly twenty years. When Anna was eight months pregnant, having lost custody of her older children, she found and was trying to enroll in a one-year residential program for women and children. Anna had missed multiple appointments because she didn't have transportation. When she called the program to explain, Anna recognized the voice on the other end of the line as a person she knew but hadn't seen in years. "Where are you? I'm coming to get you." That astonishing coincidence and the car ride that followed made it possible for Anna to begin her journey of recovery.

Anna is now the director of a "peer respite" program in Charlotte, North Carolina. A peer respite provides a safe space for people experiencing mental health crises. There are different models of peer respite. Anna's respite is organized and run by peers, not by non-peer supervisors. It is based on a successful model from Massachusetts. There are beds for short stays (up to ten days in Anna's program), but there are no clinical services or restrictions on movement. In these ways, a respite is basically the opposite of a locked psychiatric hospital or unit. Anna describes it as a bed-and-breakfast-like environment.

Peer respites are not appropriate for people in truly dangerous situations, who may need involuntary hospitalization, but respites provide a nonrestrictive, supportive, residential option. Clients at the respite are asked up front what they hope to get out of their stay. The staff are guided by those goals, not some preset vision of how recovery should look. Anna explains:

> *It's all driven by the person. . . . We're not fixers. We don't have that power. But we can walk with you as you're working on whatever, or we can sit with you if you want to . . . just safely share what you're going through and vent without fear that you're going to be labeled or given medication or forced to go into treatment. Like it's just a safe space to be who you are, where you are, and [we're] not gonna try to change any of that. Our biggest tool is sharing our experiences and holding space, creating space for people to just be. So it's just a very different healing approach.*

To meet a client where they are, it helps to have been there. How else could you even find them? Anna's respite is fully staffed "with people who have variations of lived experience around distress." Relationships are the key.

Shortly after the respite opened, Anna told me, a person of color with hallucinations came seeking services. Call him Eugene.[*] A White male staff member saw a rolled cigarette and accused Eugene of having marijuana in the respite, which is prohibited. The accusation went something like this: "You got to get out of my area. You can't have that in here." Things escalated quickly. Soon, Eugene was cursing, screaming, and even threatening violence. He was afraid that the staff member would call the police. He wasn't worried about a drug charge—the cigarette wasn't

---

[*] Not his real name.

marijuana. But Eugene had been badly injured by law enforcement in the past and, as Anna put it later, lived in "a loop of that trauma." He had already been banned from many county resources. Eugene yelled that he should "just go fuck them [i.e., the respite staff] up, you know. They're gonna call the police and ban me anyway."

If you think you know how this story ends, you don't.

At the height of the confrontation, Eugene called Anna, whom he had known and trusted for years. Anna had seen other providers misinterpret Eugene's "assertive" behavior as "aggressive." Anna didn't know it at the time, but the respite staff member who first confronted Eugene was also working part-time at a shelter that had banned him. That history exacerbated the situation. Anna also explained to me that Eugene did use marijuana to counteract side effects of his psychiatric medications, but he didn't do it at the respite because he knew it was against the rules.

On the phone, Anna was able to calm Eugene down and reassure him that no one was going to call the police. Then Anna asked essentially the same question that saved her own life: "What do you need right now? What do you need from us?" Eugene answered, "I need different staff here." So, Anna sent two new people to sit with him until the next shift arrived. Needless to say, Eugene wasn't arrested or banned. On the other hand, the staff member who overreacted that day no longer works at the respite—he wasn't a "good fit," Anna explained.

In contrast, Anna told me about another early visit that shows the limitations of the peer respite model. A mother brought her adult child to the respite and they created a plan that seemed like a good fit for everyone. The director at the time took the guest to the grocery store and the person bought a box of matches. "What are the matches for?" the director asked. "I smoke and hide it from my mom." Later that day, the guest lit their mattress on fire and refused to leave the room. They had to be physically removed. No one was hurt, but the room was damaged. The executive team came together and talked it through. They hadn't known that the guest had attempted suicide earlier that same day, which might have changed the plan or led the respite not to take on that client. The person had to be hospitalized for a time. Another learning point was to be wary of potential coercion—the peer respite model doesn't work for everyone and definitely doesn't work when people are pressured into it.

***

Recognizing that people with mental illness are in fact people has radical implications for inpatient care. The top priority should be expanding humane and cost-effective inpatient alternatives, like EmPATH units, crisis centers, and peer respites. Second, the horrendous conditions of facilities like Bryce can never be allowed to return. Those who call for "more beds" in psychiatric hospitals should have to explain how exactly they will defy the well-worn historical pattern of underfunding, neglect, and outright abuse. Finally, a person should be detained involuntarily for treatment only if there is a clear, imminent threat of physical harm to self or others and less intrusive options fail. Implicit in the phrase "civil commitment" is detention by force and/or threat of force. This option must be a last resort.

Recall Jesse Mangan's story of hospitalization with anorexia. Twenty years later, a Canadian podcast wanted to interview Jesse about his experiences. The idea set off a debate among the producers. Because Jesse had a serious mental illness, they told him, they weren't sure they could trust his consent. The producers decided to go forward with the interview, explaining that it was because Jesse was diagnosed with anorexia. "If it had been bipolar disorder, we wouldn't be able to ethically interview you." A shocked Jesse said something like this: "You realize I'm making my own podcast whether or not you interview me, right?" And he did.

Inspired by his own experience, the first season of Jesse's podcast *Committable* explores the law, policy, and experience of involuntary hospitalization. *Committable* combines key moments from Jesse's life with expert interviews. "Who is your target audience?" I asked Jesse. "My focus is always the people who are either going through the system or fear they might be." But the most engaged demographic has turned out to be attorneys and law schools. They could obviously figure out the law on their own—it's Jesse's own story that is unique. The first episode of the podcast has over a thousand downloads.

Season 2 focuses on active policy debates in particular states. I asked Jesse if he was trying to convince people in those states to vote one way or the other. No, "my intent actually isn't to tell someone how they should vote." Rather, the goal is to present information by interviewing as many people as possible. "Given the whole background of the podcast . . . I genuinely feel like everybody deserves a choice and so I try to be very careful about not vilifying anyone or anything." But the podcast does in fact vilify one thing: forcibly depriving individuals of their right to refuse hospitalization or other treatment. The podcast isn't neutral about choice, and doesn't pretend to be.

* * *

Civil commitment is very much back in the news. The pendulum in many states and localities is swinging toward expansion (chapter 5). But sometimes lesser restrictions on liberty are sufficient to mitigate the risk of harm. Recall how Leslie's peer response team de-escalated a dangerous situation by keeping the individual away from the knife he had previously been wielding (chapter 1). Extreme Risk Protection Orders (ERPOs) or "red flag laws," share the same premise. Around twenty states authorize suspending an individual's gun rights when they pose an imminent threat due to a mental health crisis or other reason. This targeted response contrasts with civil commitment or incarceration, which would mean depriving a person of all their civil liberties at once by locking them up in a hospital or jail.

By removing the most lethal method of suicide and homicide based on specific behaviors, rather than diagnoses or symptoms, red flag laws are saving lives more efficiently than other approaches. It has been variously estimated that issuing between ten and twenty-two ERPOs prevents one suicide. In contrast, the federal categorical restriction on gun possession by individuals who have been civilly committed has been estimated to deprive hundreds of individuals of their gun rights in order to prevent one suicide. Preventing homicide is more challenging than preventing suicide because homicide is less frequent and less predictable. A 2024 systematic review of studies found that the evidence regarding the impact of red flag laws on violent crime was inconclusive. But the important point is that not every potential threat requires a total deprivation of liberty.

Which brings us back to history. There is still very little evidence that involuntary hospitalization by itself has significant long-term benefits. The alternatives discussed in this chapter are not new. Nor is the evidence supporting them. Still, in most of the country, none of these alternatives are available and, even in places that do have them, there aren't nearly enough. For example, the first peer respite opened in 1993, but there were only thirty-one nationwide in 2018. Well, at least Charlotte, North Carolina, has Anna's respite. Then I asked Anna how many beds she has. "Three," she replied. That's for the nearly three million people who live in the Charlotte metro area.

TAKEAWAYS

- Inpatient psychiatric facilities have a long history of abuse and neglect.
- Some people who experience this trauma later avoid the healthcare system altogether.
- Conditions in these institutions have improved, but involuntary hospitalization remains a traumatic experience with little to no evidence showing long-term benefits.
- Connecting people to care in the community is the way to avoid the next crisis.
- Innovative ways to improve inpatient care, and reduce the need for it, should be expanded: peer bridgers, peer respites, stand-alone crisis centers, and the EmPATH model.

CHAPTER 3

JAIL

Many of the old state psychiatric hospitals have been replaced by jails and prisons.* There are now ten times as many people with mental illness in jails and prisons as there are in state psychiatric hospitals. The three largest mental health facilities are the jails in Los Angeles, Chicago, and New York City. Altogether, as of 2016, a conservative estimate is that 380,000 people with serious mental illnesses (SMIs) are in jail or prison in the United States. The rate of mental illness in prison is roughly double (41 percent) the rate in the general population.

These statistics have multiple causes. Diagnoses like schizophrenia and symptoms like first-onset psychosis do carry a significantly increased risk of violence. But that is only a very small part of the explanation. One 2015 study estimated that curing all active psychotic and mood disorders would eliminate just 4 percent of interpersonal violence. To be sure, that 4 percent figure represents enormous numbers of violent acts and victims, but it accounts for only a small percentage of the people with mental illness in jails and prisons.

Two causes of the mass incarceration of people with SMI are that they tend to live in high-poverty, high-crime neighborhoods and have co-occurring substance use disorders. That was one implication of the landmark MacArthur study discussed in chapter 1. Indeed, after

---

* States vary but, in general, "jails" hold both defendants before trial and defendants convicted on relatively minor charges. "Prison" is reserved for defendants serving longer sentences after their convictions.

controlling for these two factors, people with mental illness were found to be no more likely to be violent during the year after a psychiatric hospitalization than similarly situated people without mental illness. About half of incarcerated people with mental health conditions are there for nonviolent offenses.

Violence prevention alone cannot explain why there are so many people with mental illness in the criminal system. What does? What happens to people with mental illness after they enter the system? And, perhaps most important, what are the ways out?

* * *

In April 2019, Alaina Jean Marie Robbins experienced a mental health crisis on a public road in Cecil County, Maryland. Robbins promptly complied with police instructions to drop her weapons, but she later struggled with the plainclothes officers, explaining that she did not believe they were actually the police. After subduing Robbins, the officers transported her to the sheriff's office. There, Robbins, a small (and at this stage, naked) woman still very much in mental health crisis, allegedly assaulted multiple police officers. None of the officers suffered any serious physical injury.

The district attorney charged Robbins with thirty-five criminal counts (yes, thirty-five), including assault, reckless endangerment, malicious destruction of property, illegal possession of a rifle, attempted escape, and possession of controlled paraphernalia. She was convicted at trial on many of these counts. However, the appellate court overturned the convictions because the state unlawfully withheld relevant evidence. Undeterred, the state had another go at Robbins. In a second trial, she was convicted of resisting arrest on the roadway, as well as five assault charges based on her conduct at the sheriff's office.

Robbins appealed again. The appellate court decided that it was compelled by law to affirm the convictions, but the court did not hold back in its criticism of the police and prosecutor:

> *The charges, trials, and resulting sentence in this case have needlessly and cruelly criminalized the acute mental health crisis that Ms. Robbins suffered on April 16, 2019, and to no productive end. . . .*
>
> *The decision to prosecute Ms. Robbins for assaulting the deputies during her stop at the Sheriff's Office at all can be viewed only as punishment for her failure to comply obediently with the officers' directives, even though . . . her reactions were a function of her mental health crisis. . . .*
>
> *This whole saga punished Ms. Robbins severely while making nobody in Cecil County any safer. What was the point, other than to punish a citizen whose mental health crisis required law enforcement officers to do their jobs? . . .*
>
> *Ms. Robbins was grossly over-charged, over-prosecuted, and over-sentenced when what she really needed was help.*

Robbins is a dramatic example of how mental illness can lead to incarceration. Most cases are much more banal. Robbins actually did commit a violent offense by using force against the police officers ("assault"). In contrast, using force is not required for a charge of "resisting arrest." And many more people with mental illness end up in jail on even smaller charges, like disorderly conduct, jaywalking, sitting on a sidewalk, or trespassing. Overall, about a quarter of people in jail are serving time for low-level offenses like these.

***

What happens in jail to a person with mental illness is almost unbelievable. Most jurisdictions require cash bail for pretrial release. A 2012 report of New York City arrests found that only 12 percent of individuals with mental illnesses made bail, as compared with about 21 percent of individuals without mental illnesses, even though bail amounts were comparable between the two groups. Every arrestee is presumed innocent, but those who cannot afford cash bail will stay in jail simply because they are poor. Thus, when cash bail is required, pretrial detention becomes routine even for minor offenses and does not depend on the individual's dangerousness or flight risk.

It gets worse. A small minority of jails provide mental healthcare, and even in those jails, treatment is usually inadequate. Often, jails administer a few inexpensive drugs for behavioral control, not medications tailored to a detainee's needs. Jails that do not drug incarcerated people with mental illness into submission frequently use solitary confinement instead. One recent report found that over 122,000 people (both with and without mental illness) were being held in solitary for twenty-two or more hours on a given day in 2019. The true number is almost certainly much higher. For example, some jails are in near-perpetual lockdown, which can approximate solitary confinement. Another recent study of prisons estimated that people with serious mental illness spend three times longer in solitary than people with no mental health problems.

Solitary confinement is recognized as torture under international law, for good reason. "Soul-ripping." That's how Ethan Frost describes his time in solitary. He goes on:

You're stripped of everything. You know, you get a mattress on the floor and that's it, you know, no blanket, no sheet, no nothing. You're in a paper gown. They just, they don't check on you. They can forget about you being down. You may get a shower. You may not get a shower.

Solitary often exacerbates mental illness. It is not surprising that one study found that jail inmates punished by solitary confinement were almost seven times more likely to engage in self-harm, even after controlling for length of jail stay, SMI, age, race, and ethnicity.

Solitary confinement is just the tip of the abuse-and-neglect iceberg. It is common for mentally ill individuals in jail, especially in solitary, to "decompensate," which means that their mental health conditions worsen. The combined effect of abuse and neglect in jail is lethal. The suicide rate in jails is nearly four times higher than the suicide rate in the general U.S. population. It would be hard to design jails to be less therapeutic and more deadly.

* * *

Criminal defendants have a constitutional right to participate in the proceedings against them. One implication of this right is that the defendant must have the mental capacity to understand the proceedings and to assist their lawyer. This is called "competency to stand trial." Competency is distinct from "insanity." Competency is evaluated during the criminal proceedings, whereas an insanity defense is based on the defendant's state of mind at the moment of the alleged offense. A person may have been legally "sane" when they acted, but nonetheless be legally "incompetent" when they come to court. The reverse (insane then, competent now) is also possible. Indeed, only competent defendants can raise the insanity defense or make any other critical decisions regarding their case. The most seriously ill defendants will never have that option because their criminal cases cannot move forward.

Requiring competency is essential for fair criminal proceedings, but it has become a black hole for thousands of individuals with mental illness. In many jurisdictions, there is a long delay in obtaining an initial competency evaluation, then another long delay in receiving services to restore competency if it is found to be lacking. "Restoration services" can include not just traditional mental healthcare services like medication and therapy, but can also include instruction on court proceedings and working with a lawyer. The goal is not recovery or good mental health, but merely sufficient understanding of the proceedings to move forward with the case.

A defendant can be held for restoration services only for "a reasonable period of time." If after this period there is no realistic prospect that the defendant will ever be competent to stand trial, the state must release them or initiate proceedings to move them to a psychiatric facility. Many states do not set time limits for restoration; other states allow years. As a result, defendants with competency issues can easily end up spending more time in jail than they would have if they had pleaded guilty at the outset.

Take, for example, Joshua Marsh. In January 2022, Marsh, barefoot and without a coat, refused to leave a grocery store in Grays Harbor County, Washington. Police issued a trespass citation and noted that Marsh's speech was "nonsensical." The police came back to the store again after Marsh climbed into someone else's pickup truck. This time Marsh was arrested for allegedly assaulting the police officers. Marsh was lucky to get a competency evaluation a month later. He was found incompetent, but he then had to wait six months in jail, receiving no treatment, before he was transferred to a psychiatric facility. He was still in that facility in Fall 2022. If Marsh had been competent and allowed to plead guilty, he would have long since been released.

This is not a new problem. As part of Washington's settlement in 2014, the state agreed to provide competency evaluations within fourteen days and, if needed, to begin restoration services within seven days after that. Eight years later, in 2022, only half of defendants were getting evaluations on time, and less than 10 percent were receiving restoration services on schedule. Marsh's case appears to be typical, not exceptional.

The situation is even worse in other states. By 2017, lawsuits alleging unconstitutional delays in providing restoration services had been filed in at least a dozen states. For example, Alabama agreed in a 2018 settlement to reduce delays for inpatient evaluations and treatment. Over three years later, the judge found that wait times had "barely improved at all." The average wait for evaluation and treatment was 282 days in one recent month and 155 days in another.

Prolonged pretrial detention of individuals, particularly those with mental illness, is unfair and inhumane. People remain in jail because they are sick and poor. Most jails provide no mental health treatment. Individuals with questionable competency wait long periods for evaluation and treatment. The endless delays and harsh conditions in jail put tremendous pressure on criminal defendants to plead guilty—which 90 percent to 95 percent do—perhaps believing that conditions will be better in prison.

* * *

Having a mental illness is not supposed to be a crime. In 1962, the U.S. Supreme Court in *Robinson v. California* overturned a California statute that made it a crime to be addicted to narcotics. The Court explained that while the government may criminalize the *conduct* of using narcotics, the government may not criminalize the mere *status* of being an addict. It is "cruel and unusual" to punish anyone for a condition they cannot control. Though *Robinson* was only about addiction, the Court in that opinion expressly stated that the principle applies to mental illness.

Why, then, are so many people with mental illness in jail and prison? The facts of the *Robinson* case show one critical limit to its holding: Robinson himself admitted to using narcotics in the past, so the state could still prosecute him for that conduct. The subsequent "war on drugs" has had a disproportionate effect on people with mental illness, who are more likely to use illegal substances. But the problem is much bigger than drugs alone. Mental illness often leads to law enforcement involvement. *Robinson* left the door open to punishing any behavior associated with mental illness.

Until recently, two legal doctrines protected people with mental illness against unfair criminal punishment.* The first doctrine is the more famous one: the insanity defense. The second doctrine is the intent requirement, also known as mens rea—for many offenses, the government must prove that the defendant had a particular state of mind at the time of the offense. It is not theft to pick up someone else's book by accident, but it is theft to do so intentionally. The Supreme Court in 2006 and in 2020 reconsidered how these two doctrines apply in the case of mental illness.

Clark v. Arizona is a good example of mens rea. In 2000, Eric Clark shot and killed a police officer in Flagstaff, Arizona. Clark was convicted of first-degree murder, which required that the jury find beyond a reasonable doubt that Clark "intentionally or knowingly" killed *a police officer*. It was undisputed that Clark suffered from paranoid schizophrenia at the time of the shooting. Clark presented expert testimony that he believed "aliens" were impersonating government agents and were trying to kill him, and believed bullets were the only way to stop the aliens.

This expert testimony was offered to show that Clark intended to shoot an alien, not a human police officer—in other words, to show

---

* Competency to stand trial is a prerequisite for every criminal defendant, not just defendants with mental illness. Competency is a *procedural* right, unlike the *substantive* doctrines of insanity and mens rea discussed in the text.

that Clark lacked the required mens rea. If the testimony were believed, it should have led to an acquittal on the first-degree murder charge. However, Arizona law allowed psychiatric testimony only as part of an insanity defense. That defense failed. Clark ran away after the shooting, so he was sane enough to know that the shooting was morally wrong (or so the jury may have believed). The U.S. Supreme Court upheld as constitutional both Arizona's rule disallowing mental health testimony as to mens rea and Clark's conviction.

Effectively, *Clark* singles out mental disabilities for unfavorable treatment. Suppose Clark had no mental illness but instead had poor eyesight. He would have been allowed to introduce evidence from a vision expert stating that Clark was so nearsighted he did not know he was shooting a police officer. The purpose of the insanity defense is to protect people with mental illness from unfair punishment. It is therefore ironic that Arizona and the Supreme Court cite the availability of the insanity defense as a justification to prevent mentally ill defendants from challenging mens rea when that argument is available to non–mentally ill defendants.

Clark held that a state could allow expert psychiatric testimony for the insanity defense alone, but it prohibited considering the very same evidence for any other purpose. The Court in *Clark* left open the question of whether the U.S. Constitution requires states to recognize an insanity defense. The Court in 2020 answered that question "no." Kansas's law was just the reverse of Arizona's: A defendant could introduce psychiatric evidence only to show that an element of the offense (like mens rea) was missing. Kansas had eliminated its insanity defense, so that door was closed. In *Kahler v. Kansas*, the U.S. Supreme Court held that Kansas did not violate the Constitution by eliminating the insanity defense. Thus, the constitutionally permissible scope of criminal liability for people with mental illness is expanding rapidly. After *Clark* and *Kahler*, a person with mental illness can be convicted of a crime even if they lacked the required state of mind, even if their action was caused by their illness, even if they had no control over their action, and even if they did not know their action was wrongful.

At oral argument in *Kahler*, Justice Stephen Breyer presented the lawyers with this hypothetical: In the first case, a person with mental illness falsely believed they were killing a dog, not a person (a visual hallucination, as in *Clark*); in the second case, a different person with mental illness killed another person because he believed a dog had ordered him to do so (an auditory hallucination). Of course, the content of a hallucination does not affect culpability. Breyer therefore asked: Why does Kansas punish one case but not the other? The lawyers admitted that was true but provided no good answer to Breyer's question. Breyer could have followed up with: What's the rationale for Arizona doing precisely the opposite? There is no good answer to that question either.

At the end of the day, the Court has made clear that the government can criminally punish any behavior caused by a symptom of mental illness, even if no reasonable person would blame the defendant. If mental illness causes criminal conduct, as many people believe, then the disease is to blame for criminal conduct, not the person. The *Robinson* principle, that the government cannot punish a person for having a mental illness, is a dead letter.

These new cases require new terminology. Some advocates and academics have argued that the traditional term "criminal justice system" is not accurate, because the system is not designed to dispense "justice." Its many structural flaws include racial disparities, over-criminalization, and draconian sentences. The term "criminal legal system" is sometimes offered as a more accurate alternative label. That still gives the system too much credit. Actions caused by mental illness cannot justly be considered crimes, but that's exactly how the system treats them. At least with respect to defendants who acted due to their mental illness, the term "legal punishment system" is more appropriate. The system inflicts punishment without culpability.

Arguably, even the word "punishment" gives the system too much credit. The most common justifications given for criminal punishment are rehabilitation, retribution, deterrence, and incapacitation. The long sentences and harsh conditions in jail and prison demonstrate that rehabilitation is no longer a goal of our system. Retribution, in turn, requires that the defendant be morally responsible for the misconduct. A defendant is not responsible for conduct caused by their mental illness. Rather, society is responsible for failing to provide adequate treatment. The second justification, deterrence, also falls flat: The threat of punishment cannot cure mental illness. So an act caused by mental illness cannot be deterred in the normal way. That leaves incapacitation. On its own, incapacitation cannot justify the mass incarceration of people with mental illness. They just don't pose that significant a threat to public safety. Also, incapacitation without culpability is prevention, not "punishment."

* * *

Notwithstanding the Supreme Court's decision in *Kahler*, most states have chosen to retain an insanity defense. The insanity defense continues to capture the popular imagination, but the defense has a negligible effect on the number of people with mental illness trapped in the legal punishment system. Fewer than 1 percent of criminal cases involve the insanity defense, and it succeeds in less than a quarter of those cases. Maybe the problem is that the insanity defense is too narrowly defined? Unfortunately, a more expansive definition of insanity is unlikely to have any impact on the tragically high number of people with mental illness in jails and prisons. We know this from a judicial experiment in the District of Columbia.

In the case *Durham v. United States*, insanity was Monte Durham's only defense to the crime of "housebreaking." Before the alleged offense in 1951, doctors at a psychiatric hospital had twice diagnosed Durham with a "psychopathic personality" and once with "psychosis." In other contexts, Durham had twice been declared to be of "unsound mind." For his insanity defense to succeed, Durham had to show (1) that he was mentally ill and (2) that, at the time of the alleged offense, he was either (a) unable to tell the difference between right and wrong, or (b) impelled to act by an instantaneous and irresistible impulse. The trial court rejected Durham's insanity defense on the ground that he had failed to show either option (a) or (b).

On appeal, Judge David Bazelon* seized the opportunity to expand the definition of insanity. Specifically, Bazelon redefined the insanity defense as follows: "A person is not responsible for a criminal act if the act was the product of mental disease or mental defect." Under this new "product test," the state could not punish a person for something they did *because of* their mental illness. This new test reserved criminal punishment for actions caused by an exercise of free will. Actions caused by a mental illness were not crimes. The product test is a logical implication of the *Robinson* principle: If it is unconstitutional to punish a person for having a mental illness, then it should be equally unconstitutional to punish actions caused by the illness.

Eighteen years later, a second panel of the same appellate court ended the "product test" experiment in *United States v. Brawner*. A disappointed Judge Bazelon observed in a concurring opinion that his product test had "produced very little change at all." And while Bazelon joined the majority in adopting a replacement formulation, he had little hope that the replacement test would do any better. Under the replacement standard, an insanity defense would succeed only if the defendant lacked the mental capacity "to conform his conduct to the requirements of law."

This relatively minor change didn't matter either. Research has shown that jurors reach pretty much the same results regardless of the specific insanity definition. Changing the words of the insanity defense has little impact for an even more important reason: Even defendants with serious mental illness almost never raise the defense.

There are enormous practical reasons *not* to raise the insanity defense. Unlike with a prison term, persons found not guilty by reason of insanity (NGRI) are detained indefinitely, and they are only released if they improve clinically and are no longer considered dangerous. John Hinckley Jr. is a famous and extreme example: He tried to assassinate

---

* Judge Bazelon was a giant in mental health. The name of the Bazelon Center for Mental Health Law, a leading national advocacy organization, honors the judge's legacy of "watershed decisions" that "pioneered the field of mental health law." As we'll see, *Durham* turned out not to be one of them.

President Ronald Reagan, was found NGRI,* and was not fully released for over four decades. For individuals with severe and intractable mental illness, a "successful" insanity defense can result in what amounts to a life sentence, albeit in a hospital instead of prison.

Raising the insanity defense is risky for another reason. Defendants who raise the insanity defense and fail are punished more harshly than similarly situated defendants who do not raise it. This is broadly consistent with the common misperception that many criminal defendants abuse the insanity defense to escape punishment by faking mental illness. Jurors and judges who suspect that a defendant pursued this cynical strategy apparently add punishment for the attempted fraud.

* * *

Prison can be unspeakably cruel for inmates with mental illness. Jamie Lee Wallace ended his short and troubled life a hero. In 2014, Wallace agreed to be a named plaintiff in lawsuit alleging that the Alabama Department of Corrections (ADOC) violated the Eighth Amendment prohibition on cruel and unusual punishment by providing inadequate mental healthcare. Adding one's name to a complaint may not seem heroic, but consider the circumstances.

As a prisoner, Wallace was dependent on ADOC for all his basic human needs. By publicly challenging ADOC in this way, Wallace knew he would become a target for retaliation. He was already extraordinarily vulnerable. Wallace had a major physical disability that required him to wear adult diapers. He also had serious mental disabilities, including attention-deficit hyperactivity disorder (ADHD), bipolar disorder, and paranoid schizophrenia.

Wallace's mental health problems began early. He first saw a psychologist at age six. One of Wallace's elementary school teachers wrote that he was "often verbally aggressive," but also that he "always wanted to be accepted by the other students" and could be "very thoughtful and

---

* Public outrage over the Hinckley verdict led to nationwide legal reforms designed to curtail the insanity defense. As with the earlier attempt at expansion by Judge Bazelon, these reforms had essentially no practical effect.

generous." In 2009, at age sixteen, Wallace shot and killed his mother during an extreme mental health crisis. He had just been released from a psychiatric facility on a dramatically new medication regimen.

The state charged him as an adult. Unable to post the $138,000 bond, Wallace spent the next two and a half years in jail. Eventually, the judge found Wallace to be competent and allowed him to withdraw his insanity defense and to plead guilty, over his lawyer's objections. Wallace told the judge at sentencing: "I'd like to get twenty-five [years in prison], because simple fact is, I have been waiting so long. I can't wait for no more sentencing or nothing."

That might have been the last thing we ever heard from Wallace. Instead, Wallace agreed not only to join the lawsuit against ADOC, but to be the very first witness on the first day of trial, December 5, 2016. His testimony was damning. The prison provided woefully inadequate mental health treatment. Wallace spent most of his time in isolation (solitary confinement), decompensating. When he was alone, he often heard his dead mother's voice, which led to self-harm. Wallace had been on suicide watch more than sixty times.

Wallace described misconduct that went well beyond mere neglect. One time when Wallace was in distress, a guard offered him a razor blade and said, "You want to kill yourself? Here you go. Do it with this." Wallace also testified that when he requested mental health treatment on a different occasion, that guard "drug me out my cell and run my face in my own feces, man."

During Wallace's testimony, he became so agitated that the judge suggested he stand up. Later, the judge called a recess and moved proceedings out of the intimidating courtroom and into the quiet of the judge's chambers. Wallace said multiple times that he wanted to stop ("I'm gone, man."), but he pushed forward each time with encouragement. The judge was so alarmed by Wallace's mental state that he asked for a full report on his condition and what was being done about it.

Back in prison, Wallace died by suicide just ten days after testifying. Alabama could not keep even this one person safe. Wallace's testimony and death were critical to the judge's finding that Alabama violated the Eighth Amendment prohibition on cruel and unusual punishment by providing "horrendously inadequate" mental healthcare in its prisons. The one person who spoke at Wallace's memorial service called him, without exaggeration, "a martyr."

Alabama's prisons may well be the worst in the country, but the problem of inadequate mental healthcare in jails and prisons is pervasive and persistent. In 1994, a federal judge held that California violated the Eighth Amendment by failing to provide adequate mental healthcare in prison. California failed to correct the situation for so long that in 2011, the courts took the extraordinary step of setting a mandatory prison population limit for California. Defiant almost beyond belief, California came into technical compliance mostly by housing certain types of new inmates in jails instead of prisons, because jails were not covered by the court order.

* * *

The legal punishment system is unredeemable. In the short term, there is no realistic possibility of correcting the doctrinal and structural flaws that brutally punish thousands of people for having a mental illness. The best path forward is *around* the system, not *through* it. It is a humanitarian imperative to reduce the number of people with mental illness falling into the legal punishment system.

The first thing to recognize is that most mental health crises do not require a law enforcement response. Specialized crisis response teams not only reduce police killings; as explained in chapter 1, such teams can also radically reduce unnecessary trips to jail. Take, for example, San Francisco's *peer-led* Street Crisis Response Team (SCRT). During its first two years (from November 2020 to November 2022), SCRT handled over fourteen thousand crisis calls and engaged with people in crisis over seven thousand times—"Each engagement represents an instance that would have received a law enforcement response prior to the implementation of SCRT." In well over half of cases, the crisis was resolved at the scene and the client remained safely in the community. Most of the other engagements resulted in connecting clients to services in the community or in the hospital.

Non–law enforcement crisis response teams do not exist in most places. And even in places with crisis teams, some situations will still require a police response. Trying to understand, I suggested to SCRT peer supervisor Vania Mendoza that surely police must be sent whenever there is a weapon present. No, she explained, "all of our folks have a weapon," because they are unhoused and need to protect themselves. Police respond only if the person in crisis is "actively using or brandishing a weapon." Note the tragic irony: Police are needed to defuse a situation created in part by the city's failure to protect its unhoused residents.

Perhaps sending an unarmed team to deal with an armed person experiencing a mental health crisis strikes you as foolhardy and dangerous. It is neither. Vania could remember only two incidents—out of literally thousands of calls—where a team member was either injured or felt a threat of serious harm. That's consistent with the experience in other jurisdictions. Oregon's pioneering CAHOOTS program has operated for over thirty years without a single serious injury to a staff member (see chapter 1).

Even when a police response is required, a crisis response team can serve in a co-responder or backup capacity. This happens routinely in San Francisco. After defusing the immediate threat, police can pass the torch to the crisis team. That handoff drastically increases the chances that the individual will stay in the community and get connected with resources. Without a specialized crisis response team as backup, police may be forced to choose between two bad options: an overcrowded emergency department or jail.

There should be a third option for police (and for crisis teams as well). An independent crisis center provides short-term, emergency care for people in a mental health crisis. Care is voluntary; no one is detained or medicated against their will. A person can walk in on their own or be dropped off by family, law enforcement, or a crisis team. No matter how the person arrives, a peer counselor meets them at the door. Medical staff assess the person and recommend treatment, if appropriate. Critically, the center works with the patient to make a discharge plan, which can address not just outpatient psychiatric treatment, but also other critical needs, like housing. A person typically stays less than twenty-four hours, but individuals with greater needs can stay up to seven days. The model works. During its first sixteen months, the first crisis center in Alabama kept 255 people out of jail and 954 people out of emergency departments.

People experiencing an acute psychotic episode should be provided mental healthcare services, not taken to jail. To be sure, some people with mental illness intentionally commit crimes while fully in control of themselves. They should be held accountable for their actions on the same terms as anyone else, including being arrested and charged. What happens next is the problem.

Jail is a terrible place for a person with a mental illness. Most jails lack meaningful mental health treatment. Many jails rely instead on inappropriate medications and solitary confinement to manage behavior. Conditions in jail are already harsh for everyone, and other forms of abuse and neglect are common. The result for inmates with mental illness is very often decompensation—mental health symptoms get worse.

Eliminating cash bail for everyone should be part of the solution. No one deserves to be punished before being convicted. The legitimate reasons for pretrial detention are to ensure attendance at subsequent court hearings and to protect the public against crimes committed before trial. Jurisdictions that have moved away from cash bail—like New Jersey in 2017—have seen dramatic reductions in pretrial jail populations with no spike in violent crime or failures to appear. The current system of cash bail needlessly punishes people for being poor. Pretrial detention very often cuts off access to community mental healthcare and support.

Bail reform does not mean everyone charged with a crime is released before trial. Violent offenders and those likely to fail to appear in court will remain in jail. The vast majority of people with mental illness in jail are not violent. Recall that only 4 percent of interpersonal violence is attributable to psychotic and mood disorders. On the other hand, defendants with mental illness who are released from jail are less likely to appear in court than defendants without mental illness. The reasons are usually innocuous: People forget the court date, do not have transportation, cannot miss work, or must stay home with a child or other family member. Targeted reminders of court dates and free rides can reduce, but not eliminate, failures to appear with dramatically lower costs than incarceration. One way or another, many defendants with mental illness must decide whether to plead guilty or go to trial. Lucky defendants will have a third choice: a dedicated mental health court, where the focus is on recovery, not punishment.

Ohio judge Joyce Campbell designed and launched one of the nation's first mental health courts. There were no models at the time, so she brought together police, prosecutors, defense attorneys, mental healthcare providers, and the National Alliance on Mental Illness. If she were to start again today, she would include someone with lived experience: "That's best practices." After qualifying for the court, the first question at intake is: "What do they need?" Judge Campbell estimates that 90 percent of the people entering the program are not receiving treatment at that time. That changes on day 1, with linkage to psychiatric care, therapy, and peer support. Recognizing that treatment can succeed only when basic needs are met, the program also provides everything "from transportation to food to housing." At regular check-ins, Judge Campbell is "a little kinder, a little more patient" than on her other dockets. But there is accountability.

Mental health court is not a social services program. The fundamental purpose is to divert out of the criminal system defendants whose misconduct resulted from mental illness. That excludes, in Judge Campbell's words, "criminals that just happen to get a mental health diagnosis." At intake, after assessing need, the next question is: "What can we give them so that they can avoid a conviction?" Remarkably, over 90 percent of participants successfully complete the intensive two-year program. Judge Campbell dismisses the charges and seals the record. Not only have mental health court graduates avoided jail and prison, they have avoided a criminal record that would have limited their employment opportunities for the rest of their lives.

More than two decades later, Judge Campbell is still running the mental health court:

> *There's nothing I do that's better than that docket. When I see someone come in and their life is a disarray, and they're many times angry, and they walk out a year and a half, two years later, and they're back*

to being who they were meant to be. And they're healthy, and they're happy, and they're reunited hopefully with family and friends. That's the best paycheck in the world.

Amy Griesel was one of the first graduates of the felony mental health court in Spokane, Washington. Severe trauma, substance abuse, and paranoid schizophrenia led Amy to attempt to kill herself by fire. She was charged with arson. Amy was given the option to have her case removed from the general criminal court and transferred to the newly constituted "mental health court." This entailed a two-year intensive outpatient treatment program under strict conditions and close supervision by the judge. Amy resisted the program at first, but ultimately succeeded and avoided prison time.

Amy was not satisfied with her own success; she wanted to help others. She volunteered to be a mentor for other participants in the program. She quickly realized that she had found her "calling." She writes: "Walking alongside clients, I know I am a living model for them as I am proof that a person struggling with mental health issues and substance abuse CAN recover with help and support." Amy has since broadened her peer work beyond mental health courts. She has become a powerful voice in state government, advocating for peer work and creating new programs.

Incarcerated people with mental illness are also working to help one another. In 2012, Pennsylvania piloted a certified peer specialist program in six correctional facilities. The benefits observed within the institutions included fewer rule violations, reduced need for and use of solitary confinement, improved communication between staff and inmates, and fewer gaps in service. Peers sometimes even lead de-escalation efforts. Peers, in turn, have a meaningful work opportunity and gain skills and qualifications that may be useful after release. Perhaps most important, peer programs like this have been shown to reduce recidivism. There are now hundreds of certified peer specialists in Pennsylvania correctional institutions.

Reentry services are designed to help prisoners reintegrate into the community so that they do not end up back in the legal punishment system. Until recently, a significant barrier to successful reentry was money:

Medicaid would not pay for services in correctional institutions. That is starting to change. States can now apply for a waiver to start providing reentry services prior to release. As of August 2024, the federal government had approved eleven applications, and thirteen more applications were pending. Finally, there will be a real opportunity for advance planning and coordination with resources in the community, though the fate of these waivers is uncertain under the Trump administration.

* * *

Policymakers have other tools to increase public safety while maximizing the rights of people with mental illness. Temporary confinement alone is a blunt and largely ineffective strategy to reduce violence, either to self or others. In contrast, treatment with medication and therapy have been shown to work. Providing outpatient treatment options, first on a voluntary basis and later, if necessary, on an involuntary basis, can promote meaningful recovery and simultaneously prevent harm to others. As one researcher states, "there is also a need for more holistic approaches to maximize recovery and prevent violence, such as a combination of individual and group-level interventions, risk assessment and appropriate safety planning, in addition to pharmacological treatment (e.g., antipsychotic medication)."

TAKEAWAYS

- Hundreds of thousands of individuals with mental illness live in jails and prisons.
- Many of them may deserve criminal punishment, but many do not.
- Legal doctrines like competency, insanity, and intent allow for prolonged detention, without criminal responsibility.
- Either way, jails and prisons provide inadequate mental healthcare.
- The legal punishment system is unredeemable; diversionary mental health courts, including peer support, are promising workarounds.

CHAPTER 4

OUTPATIENT

"How do your experiences impact your work?" That was the core question during nearly every interview conducted for this book. People spoke with remarkable candor about deeply personal experiences, including childhood trauma, substance use, and time in jail and prison. I did not ask about diagnosis. Some of them mentioned medication, but many mentioned neither medication nor diagnosis. More than one subject acknowledged that they met the criteria for a particular diagnosis, but they chose not to use it because they didn't "identify with the word." Even among those who mentioned a diagnosis, that word barely scratched the surface of their unique journeys.

Jails and prisons can ignore these differences. These institutions lock people into nearly identical boxes with little regard to the lived experiences of each. That's not true in the community. One size does not fit all. The diversity of individual needs and our decentralized healthcare system mean that there are far too many community treatment models to cover in a single book, let alone one chapter. One commonly used simplifying metaphor is a staircase, where the most intensive interventions are at the top step and the least intensive are at the bottom.

This chapter describes the long-standing inadequacy of outpatient treatment options, then focuses on two intensive outpatient models. Though not without controversy, these treatment models show that institutionalization is not inevitable even for individuals with the most severe mental illnesses. The next chapter ("Community") outlines ways to support people in recovery with as little force and coercion as possible, near the foot of the staircase. Subsequent chapters will extend the recovery-oriented approach into other basic human needs and desires, like housing, employment, and education.

* * *

In 1971, the landmark *Wyatt v. Stickney* case established that individuals in state mental hospitals like Bryce have a constitutional right to treatment. Five years later, the U.S. Supreme Court held that incarcerated individuals have a constitutional right to adequate medical treatment so as to avoid cruel and unusual conditions. Critically, those rights do not exist outside of state institutions. The government has no constitutional duty to provide any treatment whatsoever to individuals not in its custody. As a result, uninsured people with mental illness in the community must depend almost entirely on charity and the political process, with little or no help from courts.

The political process has never been kind to people with mental illness. That didn't change with deinstitutionalization. In 1963, President John F. Kennedy optimistically signed into law the Community Mental Health Act. The goal was to create local outpatient mental healthcare centers to replace big state hospitals. The federal government never allocated enough money to turn this ambition into a reality. States did not pick up the slack. President Jimmy Carter tried to revive the idea and even secured substantial funding from Congress, but that law was quickly reversed when President Ronald Reagan took office. Community mental healthcare has never recovered.

Predictably, without a good public option, the fate of individuals who need treatment varies by race, wealth, and private insurance status. For example, Diane Wilson and I were held for a time at the same private hospital in Chicago. At my wife's insistence, I was transferred to another, even better, private hospital. My inpatient stay was covered by employer-provided insurance. Wilson, with fewer resources and no strong advocate, went to a state mental health facility less than ten miles away. Both with dubious mental capacity, we were convinced to sign papers authorizing "voluntary" inpatient treatment.

We both escaped. I was apprehended almost immediately; Wilson was eventually found severely injured, miles away. She would never fully recover. Wilson sued the state hospital. Because she had been admitted "voluntarily," however, the federal court held that the state had no constitutional duty to ensure her safety. Only if the state deprives a person of liberty must it compensate them with treatment. The state need not treat a person if it hasn't deprived them of liberty. This reasoning was foreshadowed by *Wyatt*, but the voluntary–involuntary distinction makes little practical sense. Either way, the state has assumed a custodial relationship with the patient. And patients who "volunteer" for the initial admission are generally not free later to come and go as they please. The doors are usually locked.

The Wilson case is important for at least two reasons. First, "voluntary" admissions compose nearly a fifth of patients in state psychiatric facilities. It is breathtaking to realize that the state has no constitutional duty to provide them with adequate care. Second, the case shows just how narrowly the constitutional right to treatment has been construed. The government can choose to provide no affordable care in the community, so low-income people with mental illness must scrape and beg elected officials for each dollar, year after year.

* * *

Decades of underfunding have resulted in grossly inadequate community-based treatment options, especially for people like Diane Wilson who lack private insurance or the means to pay out of pocket. In recent years, about half of adults with a mental illness report that they received no treatment. Cost is one of the main reasons they give. The federal Medicaid program is far and away the biggest source of funding for community mental healthcare, but Medicaid reimbursements for mental healthcare are so low that clinics lose money on nearly every service provided. Most psychiatrists have opted out and simply refuse to see any patients on Medicaid. Medicaid, like the U.S. Constitution, does not require states to provide any specific mental health service. The results are disastrous.

Mental healthcare is in crisis in every state for basically the same reasons. Take New Hampshire, for example. Medicaid accounts for around 80 percent to 90 percent of the state's total annual funding for public community mental health centers. This near-total dependence on a federal program outside the control of the state creates obvious problems. Yearly fluctuations in Medicaid reimbursement make it difficult for the state to plan or expand to meet growing needs. Nor can New Hampshire afford to raise salaries above the Medicaid rates to address its severe workforce shortage. In one post-pandemic year, the state had 250 unfilled positions at community mental health centers. The resulting delays for people trying to access treatment can exacerbate mental health problems and lead to more crises and institutionalizations.

Peers can help with the workforce shortage, but peers alone cannot solve it. That doesn't stop Ebony Martin from doing her best. Martin is a peer-to-peer support worker at a public community mental health center. Here's how she described her work to a local newspaper:

> *When you hear someone who's been through what you're going through, it's a different outreach. You see the light go on in their eyes. They think, "Oh my goodness, someone gets it." When someone has walked that path and gotten to the other side, they call it peer magic.*

* * *

Institutionalization is not inevitable. There are proven models to care for people in the community, even the most extreme cases. One example of a high-intensity outpatient model is Assertive Community Treatment (ACT). Designed specifically for individuals with severe mental illness living in the community, ACT employs a multidisciplinary team with twenty-four-hour availability and a low client-to-staff ratio. ACT is not just about managing difficult symptoms; the overriding goal is to help individuals achieve independence and become integrated into their communities. Services are tailored to the individual, not "one size fits all."

The ACT model was first developed in the 1970s, so there has been ample time to study it. What are the results? ACT improves both clinical outcomes and quality of life. There is overwhelming evidence that ACT reduces hospital days. Studies find positive outcomes including not just better medication adherence, but also better quality of life and functional status. About half of studies find improved housing stability, employment, social skills, and client satisfaction.

Lived experience matters. Research finds that ACT teams that include peers produce outcomes as good or better as ACT teams without peers. The most well-established effects of peers are increased treatment engagement and enhanced therapeutic relationships. A 2015 randomized study of veterans found that ACT teams with peers produced significantly greater improvement on an instrument designed "to assess patient's knowledge, skill, and confidence in health self-management." This is a clear example of how individuals with lived experience are empowering each other to reclaim their agency and move toward recovery.

Social worker Duncan Gibson leads the only ACT team in Birmingham, Alabama. One team is not nearly enough to meet demand in an area with a population of over one million people. Gibson puts the point this way: "I feel like we could have three more teams tomorrow and fill them up." The formal eligibility requirements are strict, including at least four recent hospitalizations or incarcerations, among other things. The actual requirements are even higher. The team focuses on the "sickest of the sick," because they can't help everyone who qualifies. Nearly all the team's 103 patients have treatment-resistant schizophrenia or schizoaffective disorder, which are arguably the two most severe psychiatric diagnoses. If a prospective client can phone the team for help, Gibson explains, then they are not sick enough to qualify.

ACT team member Mark Richards struggled with depression in childhood, then mania, and was eventually diagnosed with bipolar disorder. Gibson believes that "having a peer specialist on the team is crucial for the staff as much as it is for the patients." Everyone has some degree of internalized stigma toward people with mental illness, especially psychotic disorders. Having a peer in the room helps to break down that stigma. "We wanna laugh *with* people, not *at* people," says Gibson.

With respect to the clients, peers offer hope by showing that there is a path to recovery. Richards also engages with clients and helps them pursue their interests. Two clients who live in the same apartment complex both wanted exercise. Richards connected them and now the two patients walk together. In conversation, another client mentioned that he was a music major in college and wanted to get back into it. Richards and the client now have regular "jam sessions" twice a week—the client on keyboard, Richards on bass guitar.

Sometimes, there are unexpected opportunities for social connection. The ACT team found one client independent housing in a nice neighborhood. The client is an African American gentlemen who grew up Baptist, but had stopped going to church. One winter day, Gibson arrived to find a group of friendly Mormons in the client's apartment, socializing with the man and warming themselves on a break from door-to-door proselytizing. Now, they pick him up every Sunday and take him to church, which he enjoys. "They won't baptize him because he won't stop smoking, I think, or something," Gibson relays. But the Mormons do look after his soul in other ways, putting a Post-it note on the inside of his front door reminding him to read scripture every day.

An essential component of the ACT team is building relationships of trust and understanding. Richards's own lived experience connects him to the clients. One day, a landlord called the team to complain about a client-tenant acting intoxicated. Richards was the one to respond. He knew that the client was a regular, heavy drinker, but he also knew that the client was open and honest about it. So, when the client said he hadn't been drinking, Richards (unlike the landlord) believed the client and took him immediately to the emergency department. The client was quickly diagnosed with a critical case of gangrene and underwent emergency surgery. Richards's relationship with the client literally saved the client's life.

For the patients who need it most, ACT pays for itself. Studies have found that the reduction in hospitalizations associated with ACT programs lowers overall costs to the system. Keeping people out of jail also generates huge savings. Forensic Assertive Community Treatment (FACT) is version of ACT designed specifically for individuals with criminal involvement. A 2023 randomized study of a FACT program estimated a remarkable $1.50 return on each dollar spent.

Some critics argue that the intensive ACT model may feel coercive to clients, even though it is technically voluntary. For example, an ACT team member might threaten a client with involuntary hospitalization unless they take their prescribed medications. With enough pressure, convincing can become coercing. Some ACT clients may feel coerced, but the vast majority apparently do not. A large Canadian study asked clients about the *absence* of coercion with this question: "ACT staff do not threaten, bribe, or force me to do things that I don't want to do." Clients mostly agreed with that statement, with an average of 4.42 on a scale from 1 for "strongly disagree" to 5 for "strongly agree."

* * *

Some people living in the community refuse treatment for their mental illnesses, and some small fraction of them commit acts of violence. Media tends to focus on these outlier cases. Under pressure, state legislatures often pass bills authorizing *involuntary* outpatient treatment. Many of these bills are named for the victim, but "Assisted Outpatient Treatment" (AOT) is the term preferred by supporters. Some opponents object to the word "assisted," arguing that these laws authorize forced treatment, not mere assistance, and refer to these programs as "Community Treatment Orders" or "Involuntary Outpatient Commitment." Whatever these laws are called, nearly every state now has one.

The leading example is "Kendra's Law" in New York. In January 1999, Andrew Goldstein, who had untreated schizophrenia, killed Kendra Webdale. The legislature moved quickly, and the governor signed Kendra's Law in August of the same year. Under the law, treatment can be mandated only for individuals "unlikely to survive safely in the community" without treatment and whose noncompliance with treatment had resulted in institutionalizations or violence. Kendra's Law is relatively narrow: AOT laws in other states tend to have requirements that permit compelled treatment for broader sets of individuals.

The omission of one proposed limit on Kendra's Law was and is especially controversial. Kendra's Law permits the forced treatment of individuals who are fully aware of their illness, have unimpaired mental capacity, and make an informed decision to refuse treatment. The individual may have a good reason for refusing medication, such as religious beliefs or having had serious side effects in the past. Under Kendra's Law, the individual has no voice, no matter how clearly they are thinking at that moment. Failing to require mental incapacity for forced treatment may seem like a detail; it is not.

The Pulitzer Prize–winning novel *Lonesome Dove* by Larry McMurtry provides a vivid illustration. Augustus "Gus" McCrae is a larger-than-life, irrepressible former Texas Ranger. Very late in the novel, Gus takes two arrows to the leg. By the time he reaches help, Gus needs to have both legs amputated or he will die. His best friend, Woodrow Call, cannot convince him (nor did my screaming at the book!). For better or worse, Gus is allowed to die on his own terms.

The law respects Gus's right to refuse treatment. In 1978, a New Jersey court and a Massachusetts court each upheld an individual's right to refuse a leg amputation, even though death would likely follow. Like Gus, the litigants in these two cases were "stubborn and somewhat irascible" and "rambunctious and belligerent." The Massachusetts court stated the key principle: "The law protects [the individual's] right to make her own decision to accept or reject treatment, whether that decision is wise or unwise." Furthermore, every adult is presumed to have the mental capacity to make their own medical decisions.

Kendra's Law effectively eliminates the presumption of mental capacity for people with mental illness. If they have a mental health diagnosis, an individual's treatment decision carries no weight, even if made with full mental capacity. Criminal law could not tilt farther in the opposite direction, as discussed in chapter 3. Under current Supreme Court case law, a mentally ill individual can be criminally punished for conduct that was the product of the illness that occurred while the defendant lacked mental capacity. This inconsistency means that mental capacity rules are effectively a one-way ratchet to deprive people with mental illness of their liberty. Mental capacity is ignored if it weighs against forced treatment, but a loss of control can be criminally punished.

Kendra's Law authorizes a substantial restriction on liberty, with no weight given to the individual's choice, even if the choice was made with unimpaired mental capacity. To be clear, this rule applies only to individuals with mental illness. If Gus had had a mental illness, Kendra's Law could have authorized forcible amputation of both his legs against his will.

Setting to one side this philosophical argument against paternalism, a key question is whether Kendra's Law is delivering on its promise to improve outcomes. The effectiveness of AOT remains controversial more than two decades after it was first enacted. Preventing deaths like Kendra's was the impetus for the New York law, so it is somewhat ironic that Kendra's Law would not have helped Kendra. Her killer had untreated schizophrenia, but not because he refused treatment. To the contrary, the mental health system turned him away when he voluntarily sought help.

There are many studies of AOT that examine treatment compliance, engagement, hospitalization, arrest, and improvements in functioning. The three most rigorous of these studies randomly assigned individuals into treatment and control groups, then compared their outcomes. Two of these randomized controlled studies found no benefits. The third reported a reduction in rehospitalizations and observed other positive outcomes from mandatory treatment, but only if the mandate lasted longer than six months.

Studies with less rigorous methodology have generally found substantial benefits. One of the most thorough nonrandomized studies was commissioned by New York and published in 2010. It found positive effects in all the domains listed above. Importantly, New York increased funding for outpatient mental health services at the same time as it enacted Kendra's Law. This makes it difficult to determine whether improved outcomes were caused by Kendra's Law or by the increased funding.

To disentangle these effects, the 2010 study compared people receiving ACT alone with people receiving ACT under an AOT order. The study concluded that the treatment order did produce benefits *in addition to* the benefits from extra services. This finding is critical. Kendra's Law authorizes a treatment order only if the order is expected to have benefits above and beyond what voluntary options can provide. Enacting a version of Kendra's Law without providing additional resources for services is unlikely to yield significant benefits.

A mandatory treatment order under the terms of Kendra's Law cannot be justified if a voluntary approach would work just as well. Before a mandatory treatment order can be entered, the judge must find "by clear and convincing evidence" that "the proposed treatment is the least restrictive treatment appropriate and feasible." This requirement has been in the text of the statute from the beginning and remains there today. One might think that this would require a treatment order to be the "last resort," imposed only after voluntary options have failed or been deemed futile. That is not how things have turned out.

Almost immediately after passage of Kendra's Law, judges began reading "least restrictive" to mean "less restrictive." That effectively eliminated the requirement, because AOT is always less restrictive than involuntary hospitalization. In 2001, one judge even justified a treatment order under Kendra's Law on the ground that it would be a "far less restrictive and intrusive alternative than subjecting a mentally ill respondent to the criminal justice system." The existence of more restrictive options does not satisfy the plain language of Kendra's Law. The relevant question is whether any *less* restrictive option would work, not whether a *more* restrictive option exists.

This misreading of Kendra's Law has had alarming results. In one case, the judge used Kendra's Law to take away an individual's control over his own finances, because the individual was "unable or unwilling to pay his doctor bills and other bills, thereby resulting in his failure to receive medication and qualify for Medicaid." Consider for a moment the significance of the word "unable." It implies that an individual's poverty can be a sufficient basis to deprive them of liberty. That is indefensible in light of two obvious less restrictive alternatives: free or subsidized medication, which may already be available with assistance applying for Medicaid.

Judicial misinterpretation of the "least restrictive alternative" language in Kendra's Law preserves the status quo that the state is not required to offer any outpatient mental healthcare. For example, New York at any time could stop funding voluntary ACT and then use the unavailability of ACT to justify treatment orders under Kendra's Law. Underfunded outpatient mental healthcare increases the likelihood of unnecessary coercion in every state, not just New York.

Even as New York has expanded AOT, it has experimented with a less coercive peer-led alternative called Intensive and Sustained Engagement Team (INSET). The first INSET team was launched in 2017 in Westchester County. INSET offers a voluntary set of supports and peer services to individuals who meet AOT criteria. "Persistence" and "peers" substitute for "coercion" and "courts." And they work. Early experience with INSET demonstrates that many people who qualify for AOT will eventually accept voluntary treatment—as many as 83 percent in early trials. The lengthy engagement phase generally required for INSET builds "rapport, trust, and mutuality," but it does take significant time and effort. In contrast, AOT can mandate immediate treatment but without empowerment, self-determination, and self-directed treatment goals. AOT is not going away any time soon in New York, but the state legislature recently allocated more resources to expand the INSET model, recognizing that persistence without coercion can be effective even among some of the hardest to reach individuals.

* * *

Criminal trespass.

That was the charge Eric Smith's parents brought against him for being on their property without permission during a psychotic episode. Eric's former psychiatrist had told his parents that because Eric wouldn't agree to go to the hospital and because his symptoms weren't severe enough for involuntary treatment, jail was the only way to get Eric a psychiatric evaluation. After about a month in jail, including three weeks in solitary confinement, it worked. The judge transferred Eric from jail to involuntary psychiatric hospitalization.

Eric identifies this moment as critical to his recovery. Before the arrest, Eric had gone from star student to high school dropout due to mental health and substance use problems. It would take two additional hospitalizations, scores of medication changes, and a multitude of his own "baby steps" for Eric to achieve stability and success. "I would not have been able to get to that point without a strong support system, family, judge, attorney, psychiatrists, social workers, just the system in general." Eric now runs his own consulting business for individuals and families navigating serious mental health problems. He is also a commissioner on the Texas Judicial Commission on Mental Health and a member of the Schizophrenia and Psychosis Action Alliance Board of Directors.

Eric draws upon a deep well of practical wisdom. He is neither a lawyer nor a healthcare provider, but he can explain how mental health struggles feel from inside and describe strategies that worked for him. For example, his parents hid his laptop during a period in which it was exacerbating his conspiracy delusions. Often with psychosis, Eric explains, the goal is finding "the least-worst option," containing a fire that is already burning. Eric recommends that friends and family ask open-ended questions rather than make observations like, "you look angry." An individual in crisis may be thinking deeply about something as benign as the alphabet, so that a well-intentioned observation like "you look angry" feels like an accusation and an accelerant for paranoia.

For the clients with mental health diagnoses, Eric's recovery story provides hope and inspiration. He explains that each individual must set their own goals and work hard to achieve them, one step at a time. Recovery is rarely linear and will not happen overnight. Convincing individuals to continue taking medication even when they feel better is a recurring challenge. Eric described how those conversations often go: The obvious question, "What happened last time you went off your meds?" is more impactful when Eric is the one asking it. Both with respect to peers and families, Eric's lived experience gives him instant credibility. But Eric's consulting work is less well-known than his advocacy.

Eric is a leading advocate of Assisted Outpatient Treatment. Eric attributes his successful recovery to being placed into that program upon discharge from his first hospitalization. Eric credits his participation in AOT for being "ordered swiftly right back into the hospital without waiting," for the second and third times. At least he didn't have to sit in jail again. It was during this third hospitalization that the psychiatrist discussed with Eric how they had tried "pretty much every antipsychotic" and how basically only one option remained, clozapine. It would require close monitoring. Still delusional, Eric interpreted this conversation as evidence that he really was "a high-value asset" to the FBI. Clozapine has turned out to be an amazing drug for Eric. He described to me waking up "quiet and calm" within weeks of starting it.

Eric's story demonstrates that AOT can be appropriate and effective for some people. As with mental health courts, the most important variable is probably the judge. For example, after Eric's first hospitalization, he was discharged to a group home. Another resident of the group home kept drooling on Eric's folded clothing, so Eric's father took him home. At the next AOT hearing, the judge admonished Eric, explaining that leaving the group home was not allowed. But instead of ordering reinstitutionalization, the judge questioned Eric's father about his ability to care for Eric at home. The judge allowed Eric to move back home. Both in that moment and more broadly, the judge's flexibility and compassion were "absolutely crucial" to Eric's success. Eric knows other judges overseeing AOT who are much less involved and speak much less with participants and families.

I asked Eric about whether any the AOT program included peer support. Not formally, he explained, but there was lots of interaction with other people waiting for their hearings. Eric had seen many of them before in hospitals, where they were "just as nuts as I was." Eric was struck by their improvement: They were "now like more human and present." It seemed to Eric that most of the other peers also looked forward to meeting with the judge. The orange juice, donuts, and a movie in the waiting room helped.

The main criticism against AOT is coercion and force. That was not Eric's experience. Eric's judge did not use punishments to compel medication adherence. Without AOT, Eric believes he would almost certainly have experienced forced treatment in jail or in the hospital. AOT was *less* coercive. At least as perceived by Eric, his probate judge was ordering treatment only when it was the least restrictive alternative, unlike some New York courts under Kendra's Law. Another approach differing from New York's is the requirement in Texas that, to qualify for AOT, an individual must have a demonstrated "inability" to participate in "voluntary" outpatient treatment, as demonstrated by their recent actions or by a "significant impairment" in their decision-making ability.

Eric's journey shows that compelled treatment can achieve good outcomes. The debate is over whether better voluntary services could achieve similar, or even better, results. If pressed, even the strongest proponents of individual autonomy would probably recognize that some circumstances may justify compelled outpatient treatment. The director of the Birmingham ACT team, Gibson, described her frustration in not being able to extend AOT beyond six months for patients who are violent, lack decision-making capacity, and need medication to survive in the community. For patients like these, the alternatives may be institutionalization, homelessness, or death.

* * *

So far this book has been largely about reducing the number of people in mental health crisis who end up dead or institutionalized. But public policy should aim much higher—not just reducing bad outcomes, but also promoting good ones. To paraphrase Bryce Hospital survivor and peer Mike Autrey, the goal is to empower people with mental illness to "create the lives that they want." The rest of this book will take on that challenge. That recovery-oriented perspective will necessarily take us well outside the commonly accepted boundaries of "mental healthcare."

TAKEAWAYS

- Community mental healthcare is under-resourced and poorly coordinated.

- People with serious mental illness have widely disparate needs.

- Even among those with the most serious illnesses, involuntary treatment is not inevitable.

- A few need the intense monitoring and support of programs like ACT and AOT.

PART II

Recovery

CHAPTER 5

COMMUNITY

People with mental illness were empowering one another within mental institutions, and then outside them, well before the start of deinstitutionalization. One moment in particular stands out. In the 1940s, a group of ten male patients at a New York state mental hospital met regularly in what they called a "club room." After discharge, eight of them gathered together again on the outside. They began visiting patients at the hospital, both providing support and inviting patients to join the group after release. The name they chose was: "We Are Not Alone."

This self-help group of peers evolved to become Fountain House, which operates to this day in Manhattan and the Bronx. According to former board member Cyrus Napolitano, "Fountain House creates . . . a transitional environment and intentional community that supports people with serious mental illness to go back out in the world and live a full, fulfilling life." The "clubhouse" model pioneered at Fountain House has been copied in more than thirty countries and forty states, with around sixty thousand members in the United States alone.

Fountain House is an intentionally nonclinical environment. Fountain House doesn't itself provide psychiatric care, but it does provide care management to connect members with providers in the community. Members don't ask each other about their diagnoses—that would be "completely inappropriate," says Cyrus. He explains that his mental health diagnosis doesn't define him; rather, he defines himself as a brother, son, mentor, and teacher. Fountain House is, first and foremost, a place to connect and build community with other people who have had similar experiences to yours. According to one member, "the most powerful thing was peer support."

Membership and activities at Fountain House are all voluntary. Freedom and choice are top priorities. Many members need this opportunity to regain their sense of autonomy after their time in psychiatric facilities that some refer to as "total institutions" that constrain every aspect of daily living. The traditional hierarchy between providers and patients disappears at Fountain House. Clubhouse members help each other achieve a wide range of life goals, both practical and creative. There is support for artistic expression, both at the clubhouse and at an affiliate gallery in Manhattan.

Research finds that clubhouses reduce severe psychiatric symptoms and the need for psychiatric hospitalization. In this way, Fountain House protects its members' liberty while simultaneously bringing down overall healthcare costs. One internal study found substantial cost savings from reduced criminal justice involvement and increased wages. But Fountain House's real successes are not measured in dollars and cents. The clubhouse model increases quality of life and self-esteem, decreases internalized stigma, and promotes greater recovery experiences. One member told me that the clubhouse saved her life.

The clubhouse model is probably not what first comes to mind when you consider outpatient mental healthcare. You may be asking: Where are the psychiatrists? Where are the medications? Fountain House shows that a supportive community of peers can dramatically reduce the need for more expensive and intrusive medical interventions. New York state is taking note by providing $8 million in its 2026 budget to establish up to five new clubhouses.

In May 2023, the U.S. Surgeon General, Dr. Vivek Murthy, declared that loneliness is an epidemic with profound negative effects on health and well-being. This is particularly true for people with severe mental illness, who are twice as likely as other people to experience loneliness. Fountain House exists to bring "members" together to support one another. Combating loneliness is built into its DNA. Recall its original name: We Are Not Alone. Research confirms that the clubhouse model promotes a sense of unity and belonging. It is therefore not surprising that, in formulating his strategy to reduce loneliness, the Surgeon General's panel of experts included the chief research officer of Fountain House.

* * *

Mental health crises are often likened to hurricanes, and Sonny Leppala speaks from personal experience when he draws this connection. He holds a master's degree in mechanical engineering and used to work at a floor tile plant in New Orleans. "Everything was good, a lot of responsibilities, production supervisor, project engineer, a little bit of everything." Then came Hurricane Katrina. Almost overnight, he lost his job, and his rent doubled. He moved in with his sister in Helena, Alabama, but she eventually had to make the "very hard decision" to kick him out. He had developed alcohol and substance use problems, along with undiagnosed mental illness. Sonny was homeless.

Sonny sought help from the Salvation Army, which recognized mental health was an issue and connected him to a case manager at Jefferson Blount St. Clair Mental Health Authority (JBS). He made it to a JBS clinic, but his symptoms were so severe at that point that he was immediately transferred to a hospital, his first visit to a psych ward. As discussed previously, most people in psych wards are desperately trying to get out. Not Sonny. He was so afraid of being homeless again that he "put on a big show of paranoid schizophrenia." He did not actually have any delusions or hallucinations. "I was fearful of my life. It was like a defense mechanism. So I don't apologize for [fooling people] . . . it's what I felt like I had to do to survive."

During Sonny's hospitalization, staff registered him for disability benefits and placed him into a group home after discharge. He lived for about two and a half to three years at the group home. His doctor at the time misdiagnosed Sonny with major depression with psychotic features. Sonny, who now has a diagnosis of bipolar II disorder, laments the overreliance on psychotropic medications. They had me on "maybe nine medications," including "multiple antipsychotics" and "multiple antidepressants." Sonny is also highly critical of the day program he attended at the time. Some good people work there, Sonny is quick to observe, but expectations are generally way too low, and worst, from Sonny's perspective, "they're not really goal setting."

After the group home, JBS moved Sonny into an apartment in the community. Shortly thereafter, Sonny started working as a "peer bridger" to help others manage the transition from group homes to independent living. Although Sonny is extremely grateful for his apartment, he wishes the system worked better for other people. "First of all, they don't get integrated into the community. They get placed. And that's typically the place where they're going to die." A high percentage end up abusing substances. "We did the best we could, but I, you know, I just think the system didn't do enough."

Sonny thanks his own peer work for keeping him moving in a positive direction. "I'm always saying get yourself back to work, do anything . . . volunteer, all of that. Be productive, do meaningful stuff, stay out of trouble." Sonny works at the Birmingham stand-alone mental health crisis center described in chapter 2. He puts in as many hours as he can without going over the income threshold that would disqualify him from receiving public benefits. The short time period a patient spends in the facility can be transformative, Sonny explains, but progress can be sustained in the long run only by building connections in the community to avoid the next crisis. That's where Sonny focuses his energies.

Sonny is effective in this role precisely because of his experience being homeless and suffering from addiction and mental illness. "As a peer support specialist, I get to help people based on those experiences. . . . So it's like I'm taking that crap, that part of my story, and making it into something that's worthwhile and helping other people in the process." He fills a role that non-peer clinicians cannot. Peers may not be immune from stigma and self-stigma, but they are more likely to relate to, and less likely to judge, a person who has shared experiences. And he knows relapse is part of recovery.

Sonny cannot say enough good things about his own mentor and peer, Jon Brock. Jon was one of the first peer specialists at JBS. Sonny met Jon at the day program and Jon has been there for Sonny ever since, fifteen years and counting: "He met me where I was in my recovery and we just went from there." Jon provided just enough support to "empower" Sonny rather than being a "crutch." Sonny explains: "The one thing I've learned from him more than anything else was learning how to listen to other people who are going through those struggles.... I learned better how to do less ... enabling the folks ... to go on to succeed on their own."

Like many, Sonny started doing peer work early in his own recovery journey. He became a peer bridger not long after his own transition out of a group home. That work, and his work at the crisis center, have been important to his own recovery. Seeing people in crisis motivates him to take better care of himself. He becomes more proactive in his own recovery.

***

Hands Across Long Island (HALI) is an entirely peer-run organization with a range of programs including the weekday, drop-in Recovery Center. CEO Melissa Wettengel's face lit up describing a recent event:

> *We just had an open mic at the Recovery Center. And it's part of, you know, quote programming for the Recovery Center. But we just put it out to staff if anybody wants to come in. Even people who are in different divisions, you know, housing or mobile shower unit, and people just came in. And, you know, first it's like formal signups, and then people just start popping up, and it was just gorgeous, like when people can just express themselves. And you learn things about people that you didn't know. And this one's singing Kenny Rogers ... it's just a lovely, lovely thing. And when sometimes we have moments like that, I'm just like, This is why HALI's special. There's such a safe feeling here at HALI for the people who come to the Recovery Center. They just want to be here, you know. It's a place where everybody knows their name.*

Physical well-being is another major emphasis because studies show that people with SMI have substantially shorter life expectancies. A mobile primary care van visits the Recovery Center regularly. Counseling around diet and diabetes takes place, but is less fun than the healthy-ingredient cooking contest inspired by the television show *Chopped*. A lot of creative programming ideas come from the staff but suggestions by others in the community are rarely rejected.

The goal of the Recovery Center is not just to build a community and promote wellness within its walls. A broader goal is to facilitate people who want to integrate back into the community outside. A field trip to a public park or historic Long Island mansion is followed up with encouragement and transportation instructions for getting there on one's own. There are traditional support groups for emotional and relationship issues, but also more educational groups. One support group helps participants prepare advance directives to govern their care in the case of an emergency hospitalization (see "Epilogue"); another group provides instruction on how to avoid losing benefits as a by-product of gaining employment (see chapter 7). There is an entire advocacy team devoted to that critical issue. When a person is ready to talk about any specific goal, one-on-one support is available. One of the first questions asked at the Recovery Center is likely to be, as Melissa framed it: "What did you want to be when you grew up, like before all this shit happened to you?"

* * *

Private insurance is no guarantee of quality mental healthcare. I struggle just to stay on top of my own complex and changing combination of medications. There are severe shortages of psychiatrists, therapists, social workers, and other providers. Many are not taking new patients, and others have long waitlists. People with the most serious mental health problems need a team of providers not just for healthcare, but for basics like food, housing, and transportation. There is no unified mental healthcare system. Each person must put together their own team. Care coordination is essential but can be elusive.

I first received mental healthcare in my early thirties. I had struggled with an unnamed sadness—almost certainly undiagnosed depression—since I was very young. My wife urged me to talk to a therapist or a doctor, but I resisted. I was dropping balls left and right, including failing to update our license plate stickers. After a police officer pulled us over, my wife tearfully pleaded one last time for me to get help.

I started seeing Kathleen O'Grady, the therapist who would change my life. But talk therapy took me only so far. Eventually, my primary-care doctor prescribed me an antidepressant. With Caroline's and my connections, finding a great therapist and getting a doctor's appointment were easy for me. No long waiting list for the lucky and privileged.

When, to everyone's shock, the antidepressant triggered severe mania, I didn't wait days in an emergency room. I was taken by ambulance to the closest hospital, where my wife worked. She insisted that I be taken to a second hospital with a better inpatient unit. I was safely installed in the unit within a few hours.

After my first hospitalization, I had little trouble finding outpatient psychiatric care. My first psychiatrist had been my attending physician on the psych unit. He was excellent clinically, but I ended up firing him because I thought he was too paternalistic. With no hard feelings, he seamlessly referred me to another, more junior psychiatrist. I was able to persuade this second doctor to suspend my antipsychotic medication, which likely contributed to my second manic episode. I'm not sure I could have convinced my first psychiatrist to hold that drug. What we want is not always what is best for us, but my status gave me choices others would not have.

When my second psychiatrist chose to focus his practice exclusively on uninsured and Medicaid patients, I had another seamless transition. My third doctor was Goldilocks for me: senior yet sensitive. She helped me find a stable medication regime of lithium and Risperdal, which blunted the worst of the depression and kept me out of the hospital for years. But this doctor's greatest gift to me was inviting me to speak with a group of her psychiatry residents.

At that time, psychiatry residency was tilted toward inpatient care. That meant residents rarely saw patients doing well. I was able to shatter some of their stereotypes. One resident asked how I could work as a lawyer while taking mind-numbing dosages of lithium. "Excess capacity," I quipped. Caroline still cringes at the arrogance of that remark. I believed it then, and I believe the same is true of nearly everyone with a serious mental illness: We are more capable than others believe. We have to be.

My outstanding outpatient care continued, notwithstanding our move from Chicago to Alabama. There was once again a white-glove VIP handoff from one star psychiatrist to another. A senior doctor at University of Alabama at Birmingham kept me stable for a few years before introducing me to Doctor Richard Shelton. Both were excellent. Head of research, Shelton was a particularly good fit for me. He knew the literature cold and provided clear explanations. His office whiteboard was often covered with hand-drawn graphs after our appointments.

Unfortunately, my remarkable run of continuity of care didn't last forever. Shelton moved from Birmingham to Huntsville, an hour and a half north. At first, I received a letter saying I could no longer see him. There was a quick policy reversal under which remote visits were allowed, but then that policy ended and I was assigned to the medical center's resident clinic. I would be seen by a different resident doctor each year. There was an attending physician, but our conversations were so brief that I never learned her name. Taking advantage of connections, I was able to find a psychiatrist in private practice.

Even with every advantage, assembling and reassembling a treatment team has been challenging for me. Finding a therapist has been the hardest part of this process for me. Therapy requires a personal connection in addition to clinical skill. For years after we moved to Alabama, I tried and failed to find a relationship like that. Eventually, I reached out to Kathleen O'Grady in Chicago, and we reestablished our relationship.

Kathleen died late in the COVID-19 pandemic. It took about a year of failed attempts to find another therapist. I became a master of the free fifteen-minute consultation. I had multiple, full appointments with two or three different therapists, but felt like I was treading water at best. One therapist took a personal phone call in the middle of an in-office session. He did have one great suggestion though: putting together a "happy playlist" of upbeat music to listen to in periods of depression. Not intentionally, but probably not coincidentally, most of the music I select and download is pretty depressing. It's sometimes helpful to feel like music is affirming a negative emotion, but it's better not to be depressed all the time. My extended search for a therapist was possible only because I have a flexible work schedule. My new therapist does not accept private insurance at all, so I'm paying out of pocket. That is obviously not a viable option for many people with serious mental illness.

Then there are the little things, which turn out not to be so little. Pharmacies, for example. I switched back and forth between CVS and Walgreens several times before settling on a small, locally owned pharmacy. The big chains couldn't keep up with my medication changes. I kept running out of prescriptions and needing to refill the same or next day. CVS was open twenty-four hours, so I started out going there. Then CVS seemed to experience a mass exodus of staff, and the lines were ridiculous. My locally owned pharmacy has limited hours, but is better in every other way. They call when things don't make sense and deliver medications to my home automatically each month. Often, they fill and deliver new prescriptions on the same day.

Missing a dose of psychiatric medication is not like missing a dose of blood pressure medication. The negative effects are immediate: I can't fall asleep without my nighttime medications or I wake up in the middle of the night too confused to realize why. Losing sleep can trigger mania, so the anxiety of a bad night's rest carries over into the next day. One advantage of the big pharmacies is being able to transfer the prescriptions to a different city if I do forget my meds when traveling. My solution? Count out my meds each week, and never, ever, forget to pack them.

My recovery journey has also included peers. I attended a support group on several occasions. There were drinks and snacks and, once, cake for a birthday. Many participants were regulars; others were first-timers. Some were in obvious distress; most were not. At the outset, everyone read the ground rules aloud and in unison. Each person had the same allotted time period to use however they wanted, then any extra time would be spent discussing the most pressing situations. Everyone's voice counted equally. The openness and absence of judgment was exhilarating. I left in awe at the quiet grace and dignity of one participant who took their full allotment of time each week to talk about their volunteer work. No complaints whatsoever, not about symptoms, not about woefully inadequate public transportation, nothing. Here is a person with far more severe symptoms than me devoting all of their available time to helping others.

*　*　*

Each person's mental health journey is unique, and few journeys are linear. There will be ups and downs, of course, but the long-term goal of recovery is to move each person down the treatment intensity staircase, and maybe even off it entirely. Doing so reduces coercion and cost and increases independence. Due to remarkable good luck and built-in advantages, I have been able to assemble and reassemble a team to manage my own mental health in the community. Near the bottom of the outpatient intensity staircase, clubhouses, drop-in recovery centers, and support groups demonstrate the power of safe and supportive communities of peers. Everything is voluntary, and no one even asks about diagnoses. Many people with mental illness, like Sonny, attribute their ability to thrive in the community in part to the sense of purpose their peer work provides. The benefits of peer support flow in both directions.

TAKEAWAYS

- Most people with mental illness will never need to be institutionalized or subject to mandatory treatment.

- Clubhouses, recovery centers, and support groups show the power of voluntary peer support in the community.

CHAPTER 6

HOUSING

The magnitude of homelessness in the United States is staggering. Over 770,000 people were unhoused on one night in January 2024—an alarming 18 percent increase from 2023. No single housing policy change alone could solve such an enormous problem. Among unhoused people, about 25 percent to 30 percent have a serious mental illness (SMI). By comparison, only 6 percent of the overall population has an SMI. The inadequacy of mental healthcare in hospitals, jails, prisons, and outpatient settings exacerbates the problem, but treatment alone will not solve it. Stable housing is very often essential to recovery. For some people, housing must come before treatment.

Nova Honey lost her home in Portland, Oregon, because she was paranoid and hearing voices. She was diagnosed with schizoaffective disorder. Honey's yearlong search for housing was interrupted multiple times by psychosis when she wasn't able to refill her medications. She eventually found a place to live, where she receives her medications on time each month, delivered to her door. Housing alone cannot solve mental illness, but Honey's story illustrates how recovery for some is impossible without it.

Having a place to live can be transformative. As we saw in chapter 2, the director of a peer respite program defused a potentially dangerous mental health crisis by asking the individual: "What do you need right now?" When a person with SMI is unhoused, the answer is usually obvious. After people with serious mental illness are provided with permanent supportive housing, the question becomes: "What do you want?" Sometimes it's just a hot dog or a walk. Housing is very often the difference between crisis and recovery, between merely surviving and actually living. Peers can help bridge that gap.

* * *

Rafael Rodriguez describes himself as "an open book." His story begins with sexual abuse in early childhood. The resulting guilt, shame, and isolation led Rafael to comfort himself with food. By age twenty-three, he had reached 620 pounds. A doctor told him that, without surgical intervention, Rafael might not reach age thirty-five. Rafael had gastric bypass surgery the following year. He lost weight quickly but, with the underlying trauma still unaddressed, Rafael substituted alcohol for food. Later, it was cocaine.

Around this time, in 2007, Rafael's uncle was murdered. Rafael's father fell into depression and drank himself to death within a year. Rafael bonded with a new substance—heroin. At first heroin felt like the "solution": "It allowed me to exist and not live in the guilt and shame." But everything else in his life crumbled. Rafael ended up homeless on the streets of Providence, Rhode Island. He was unfamiliar with available resources and scared to enter shelters. He survived three overdoses, one of which was an intentional suicide attempt. The birth of his first child in 2009 was a wake-up call, but the path to recovery was not straight.

Rafael fell back into substance use and was arrested on a drug charge. He pled guilty and got probation. He knew he wouldn't be able to stay clean, so he asked his probation officer for help. Rafael feels lucky that he ended up placed in facilities for people with substance use, one temporary (Hope Center), then one more permanent (Opportunity House). That's where Rafael first experienced the power of what he'd come to know as peer support. It wasn't from the counselors, even though they also had lived experience. The power dynamic undermined trust. Instead, Rafael felt supported by the other residents: "On the streets we'll say that a bullshitter knows bullshit." Rafael started opening up, talking about his traumatic experiences and listening to the other residents.

Food came back into Rafael's life, but this time in a healthy way. A trained chef, he cooked for free at the facility for nine months, turning the facility's previously "terrible" food into creations that the residents actually enjoyed. This was his first inkling of how gratifying service could be. Rafael next moved to a sober home. For more independence, he moved into his own apartment. That turned out to be a mistake. Living on the street is a constant 24/7 struggle for survival. After that, the solo apartment gave him too much time to live in his own head. He slipped back into substance use and homelessness.

The birth of Rafael's second daughter convinced him that he needed to find a job. One advertisement posed two questions: "Have you experienced trauma? Would you like to support others with similar experiences?" He didn't know anything about the organization, but he applied anyway. At the interview, the staff asked him to read the following statement: "Yeah, I don't go there. That place is for those people." "What do you think about that statement?" they followed up. Rafael replied, "Well, first of all, it's a pretty shitty statement." He got the job.

That was December 2016. The organization is now known as the Wildflower Alliance. It serves primarily western Massachusetts. Rafael provides peer support to residents of Greenville, an old hotel that has been converted into single-occupancy rooms for people who have been unhoused, the vast majority with mental health challenges. When Greenville first opened, professional social workers tried to provide support. That didn't work. Residents wouldn't talk to the social workers, because the residents were afraid that talking could get them into trouble and cost them their housing.

Rafael understands. He once spent months on a waiting list to see a new therapist. At one point during the first session, he told the therapist: "I'm done. I can't do this no more." What Rafael meant was that he didn't want to keep living in the same miserable way he had been. The therapist, without asking any follow-up questions, assumed that he didn't want to keep living at all. Next thing Rafael knew, paramedics arrived and took him to a psychiatric unit, where he spent the next two weeks.

Rafael has found that shared experiences are the foundation for trust and rapport: "We're very open about our lived experience. So, we can say, 'Yeah, man, I've been homeless. Yeah, I know, I get it.'" It doesn't matter how far along a resident is in their recovery journey. There is no judgment. Rafael emphasizes that his successes and the lessons he's learned don't "make [him] better than anyone else is. Just, you know, someone was there to support me. And maybe I can be that person to support you."

Time on the street has lasting consequences, Rafael explained. The experience of having nothing leads people who become housed to fear that it will all be suddenly taken away. Rafael has himself felt that fear, so he understood exactly why one resident failed to report that their shower was backed up. The resident thought they'd be blamed and kicked out of Greenville. Only when the water started leaking downstairs did the management company enter the apartment. They found an old pipe that needed to be replaced. The resident had done nothing wrong.

Understanding this fear can lead to simple and effective solutions, illustrated by another story. The management company's new system started automatically generating written notices for residents who were two weeks late with their rent. Sometimes the rent was late, but often the rent had been paid on time and there had been a processing delay. The envelope included a large print warning about the deficiency with small print on the bottom explaining that it was not an eviction notice. Many residents were so terrified that they did not read the fine print or open the envelope. Rafael knew this feeling: "I can relate to having those fears of having letters just show up to my mailbox, and not knowing what it is, and dreading what might be the cause for them." Rafael explained the situation and advocated for two changes. Of course, the company had to fix the processing delays, but the second change might not have been obvious to someone who had not felt the fear of losing everything. Rafael persuaded the company to change the print on the envelope, so that the reassuring disclaimer about eviction appeared in big print at the top and the deficiency notice was moved to the bottom in smaller print.

A person who has been homeless may come to expect the worst and not even realize that they can ask for accommodations. In one case,

Rafael is pretty sure he kept a resident from losing their apartment. The resident really *hadn't* paid rent and had received a more formal notice that required a court appearance. Rafael asked the resident whether something was going on. That's how Rafael learned that the resident had sent his rent money to Puerto Rico to help pay for the burial of a family member. After explaining this to the landlord, they were able to negotiate a payment schedule that allowed the resident to stay in his apartment. Rafael believes that "if there wasn't support there from a peer, he would have just kept [the explanation] to himself."

The housing outcomes are not always favorable, but having a peer can still improve the process. Residents may come to feel like participants instead of victims. People are treated better in court when they come with an ally. Rafael regularly accompanies residents to court and has noticed that "things were much more clearly explained to them." Keeping individuals housed is obviously a major goal, but an even more fundamental goal for Rafael and his organization is to empower individuals to "self-determine" in all areas of their lives. That's the opposite of what politicians do.

* * *

One day on a New York City subway car, in response to a perceived threat, a White male passenger employed deadly force against a Black male passenger. There was a national media frenzy. The immediate political reactions were predictably polarized: The White passenger was either a "hero" or a "vigilante," depending on whom you asked. After several days the White passenger turned himself in to law enforcement. The mayor danced a tightrope in his public statements, ultimately (and conveniently) endorsing a grand jury indictment that split the difference between very serious and very lenient charges.

Don't worry, the mayor had a great plan for improving conditions on subways and streets: mobilize the police to forcibly remove and transport to the hospital homeless individuals who appear to be mentally ill and unable to take care of themselves. Historically, involuntary hospitalization had been reserved for people who posed an immediate danger;

ordinary self-neglect wasn't enough (chapter 2). The reason, of course, is that forced confinement is a massive deprivation of liberty.

The mayor said that his goal for expanding involuntary hospitalization was to provide individuals with the treatment they need but irrationally refuse. However, the city did not actually provide adequate mental healthcare, either in hospitals or outside of them. Nor was there enough low-income housing. As a result, critics suspected that the mayor's real goal was to make commuters and tourists feel safer and more comfortable in high-traffic areas. This suspicion was bolstered by the mayor's public statements that the new policy addressed an apparent problem we all could see.

These events in New York City happened first in the 1980s, then again in the 2020s. That's right: Every single word of this description is true for *both* time periods. The same perceived problems generated precisely the same response. Only the names have changed—yesterday's subway shooter, Bernard Goetz, was replaced by today's lethal chokeholder, Daniel Penny. The policy of expanding involuntary hospitalization failed to improve mental health or reduce homelessness, but perhaps Mayor Koch in the 1980s sincerely believed it would succeed. Mayor Adams in the 2020s had no excuse. He was a New York City police officer in the 1980s and 1990s, so he had a front-row seat to the failure of the policy he would revive forty years later.*

New York is far from alone. Many other states are considering, or have already adopted, similar measures. California has by far the most unhoused people of any state: an estimated 30 percent of the total homeless population. In response to a perceived homelessness crisis, California loosened the eligibility requirements for involuntary hospitalization. Previously, individuals had to be found unable to provide themselves with food, clothing, or shelter due to mental illness. The new standards allow for involuntary hospitalization of people unable to provide for their "personal safety" or "necessary medical care."

---

* This meets an oft-repeated definition of insanity: "doing the same thing over and over again and expecting different results."

The "personal safety" language is problematic. Is it safe for *anyone* to live on the streets? Or in shelters like the ones Rafael was too afraid to use? Is that the fault of the unhoused person, or is there inadequate public support and protection? More than a third of homeless individuals with SMI are victims of violence each year. An interesting feature of California's new law is that counties are allowed to defer implementation until 2026. That's a pretty slow response to a "crisis." The delay likely reflects the fact that there are not nearly enough hospital beds to accommodate all of the newly eligible people. As in New York, "treatment" in California looks like an excuse to move people with mental illness outside the view of tourists and voters.

To effectively combat homelessness, public policy must address its root causes. Recall that 25 percent to 30 percent of unhoused individuals are estimated to have SMI. Even within that fraction, it is important to recognize that mental illness is often caused by homelessness, not the other way around. This is particularly true of depression and suicidal thinking. Either way, over two-thirds of unhoused people are *not* experiencing serious mental illness. Obviously, other forces are at work.

The top three causes of homelessness are all economic: lack of affordable housing, unemployment, and poverty. People almost never choose to be unhoused; they just can't afford rent. In 2023, California had just twenty-four units of affordable housing available for every hundred extremely low-income households. It's not by coincidence that California has the highest rate of homelessness. Black people are more likely to be unhoused, a disparity that is driven by long-standing historical and structural racism. Between 22 percent and 57 percent of all women experiencing homelessness report that domestic violence was the immediate cause.

Both mayors of New York City knew, or should have known, these statistics, and still focused on mental illness. The reason is simple: Surveys find that members of the public (i.e., voters) rank substance use and mental illness as two of the top causes of homelessness. A tourist or commuter cannot easily ignore an unhoused person in mental health crisis yelling loudly on a subway car—like Jordan Neely, the man choked to death in 2023. People systematically overestimate the frequency of events they can remember easily. Media coverage magnifies this effect. The quiet unhoused person sitting peacefully against a wall with a hand outstretched may make no memory at all and certainly will not make the news.

It is also important to recognize that most people are unhoused for multiple reasons. Suppose a Black man has a criminal conviction for heroin possession. Heroin was the one thing he had access to that reduced the paranoid delusions associated with undiagnosed schizophrenia. Even assuming the man finds another way to control the delusions, his criminal record and race might make it impossible for him to get a job that pays enough for rent, let alone provides health insurance. The problem of homelessness cannot be solved by one fix; it will take many fixes all at once.

Mental illness does present unique housing challenges—some of which can be overcome with regular access to the right medications—but better treatment alone won't solve the problem. Many thousands of unhoused people with mental illness also need a rent subsidy, health insurance, a decent job, or all of the above. "The problem of homelessness is that people don't have housing," explains Dr. Margot Kushel, a housing expert at UCSF. "If you had all the treatment in the world and you didn't have the housing, we would still have this problem." A large-scale 2023 survey of California residents experiencing homelessness found that "even if the cause of homelessness was multifactorial, participants believed financial support could have prevented it." Note the radical study design: Ask the people with lived experience why they are homeless.

* * *

Cities do not have to wait for an individual experiencing homelessness to have a mental health crisis to lock them up. As I was writing this chapter in the summer of 2024, the U.S. Supreme Court in *City of Grants Pass v. Johnson* ruled that the government can criminally prosecute individuals with no access to shelter simply for sleeping outside. Advocates for the unhoused had argued that this amounted to unlawful status-based punishment, relying on the 1962 *Robinson* case discussed in chapter 3. Recall that the Court in *Robinson* held that criminalizing an involuntary condition like drug addiction is cruel and unusual punishment. Sleeping outside is an action, not a condition, the *Grants Pass* majority reasoned.

Justices Sotomayor, Kagan, and Jackson dissented:

> *Sleep is a biological necessity, not a crime. For some people, sleeping outside is their only option. The City of Grants Pass jails and fines those people for sleeping anywhere in public at any time, including in their cars, if they use as little as a blanket to keep warm or a rolled-up shirt as a pillow. For people with no access to shelter, that punishes them for being homeless. That is unconscionable and unconstitutional. Punishing people for their status is "cruel and unusual" under the Eighth Amendment.*

The Court's holding applies to everyone experiencing homelessness, but it will fall heavier on people with SMI because they are overrepresented among the unhoused.

* * *

OneRoof is an aptly named nonprofit in Birmingham, Alabama, that connects unhoused people to organizations that provide affordable housing. Many of its clients have mental health challenges; many do not. Jennifer Harrell is the Director of Coordinated Entry. Matching people with the right placement is the stated goal, but there isn't nearly enough housing to meet demand. OneRoof maintains a waitlist that fluctuates between 300 and 375 people, so Harrell is forced to prioritize the individuals on the list. For some people, waiting is not an option.

Even relatively short delays can lead to prolonged homelessness. Clients often come to OneRoof seeking a specific service or placement at that moment. That's generally impossible given the limited resources. One client's story illustrates what can happen next. Call him Robert. Robert had been homeless off and on for about ten years. He had been banned from multiple shelters.[*] Robert sought help from OneRoof, often

---

[*] Rafael believes that we need many more peer-run shelters. Instead of just banning disruptive people, peers would be more likely to understand and validate the person's anger and to ask, "What can we do different?"

multiple times each week. He was so disruptive that OneRoof's landlord also wanted to ban him. Robert's search for housing was interrupted by frequent detention in jail and hospital, which OneRoof would find out about only afterward. As a result, Robert had to start his housing search over again each time. Even when spots were available, it was sometimes impossible to collect all the required documentation in time. This went on for three years.

How did Robert eventually succeed in finding stable housing? Enlightened public policy? No, it was luck. Robert happened to be out of jail and out of the hospital long enough to be placed in a program with the types of intensive support he needed. Robert met with a member of the REACT team,[*] which moved him into his new apartment the very next day. He's still in the program, but that has required additional good luck. This was Robert's first time living independently. He tried cooking himself a meal and caught the apartment on fire. Robert would have been evicted, but the community rallied and raised enough money to pay for the damage.

Alabama recognized the acute housing shortage in 2012 when it created the "Housing Trust Fund" to build and maintain affordable housing in the state. Eleven years later, not a single dime had been allocated to this fund. So Jennifer at OneRoof, who has herself experienced homelessness, is constantly forced to decide which unhoused people get a place to live and which will not. Additional funding for more units is obviously needed, but money alone won't be enough. As Robert's case illustrates, the application process must be streamlined to reduce wait times, and the many parts of the "system"—including, for example, crisis centers, emergency departments, hospitals, and jails—must communicate with one another and quickly provide documentation on demand to avoid having to restart the process over and over.

* * *

The Housing First model originated in New York in the 1990s. As the name suggests, homeless individuals are quickly housed in the commu-

---

[*] Birmingham's version of ACT (Assertive Community Treatment), discussed in the next section.

nity and provided with in-home support services. Participants are not required to get sober or accept treatment in return for housing. Threshold requirements like these, no doubt well-intentioned, often exclude the people who need housing most. In other words, Housing First provides housing immediately. Residents can decide later whether to give up substances or seek mental health treatment. They keep their housing either way. Housing First is stunningly simple: Quickly provide housing to as many people as possible, then provide the supports needed to keep them housed.

More than twenty years after its creation, the Housing First model has been widely adopted and extensively researched. Not surprisingly, Housing First participants consistently experience better housing outcomes. They find housing more quickly, they stay housed longer, and they report higher satisfaction with their housing. In addition, Housing First reduces the number of emergency department visits and hospitalizations. Some studies find additional benefits, including reduced police, judicial, and welfare expenditures.

Housing First more than pays for itself. A 2022 review of six high-quality studies in the United States found a median benefit-cost ratio of 1.30 to 1. That means each dollar spent on Housing First saves the government $1.30. The primary benefits to the government are lower healthcare costs and less judicial involvement. But the total benefit of Housing First is much higher. That's because benefit-cost studies do not include the value of stable housing for participants who would otherwise be homeless, which, after all, is the primary objective of Housing First. Benefits of housing like autonomy, privacy, security, comfort, and warmth are omitted because they hard to quantify. Factoring in these direct benefits would produce an even higher benefit-cost ratio. It is remarkable that Housing First is a great investment based purely on its secondary effects, without even considering the direct benefits of being housed.

Housing First done well does not stop with housing placement. The model also includes services to keep people housed. The level of support varies dramatically depending on the needs of the clients. One of the most intensive models is Housing First + ACT (Assertive Community

Treatment, discussed in chapter 4). Recall that the clients in Birmingham's version of this program (REACT) have exceptionally severe diagnoses: treatment-resistant schizophrenia or schizoaffective disorder. That's where Robert eventually ended up.

Success for clients in this population is measured on a different scale. Rick Gish is the Housing Coordinator for the Birmingham REACT team. I asked him whether clients ever "graduate" from the program into independent housing. A few do leave, he explained, but they almost always move into another supported housing program with stepped-down services, not into unsupported private housing. A little later in our conversation, Rick offered an example of "graduation" *within* the REACT program. At the outset, some clients need to be seen every day for help with their mental health problems. As clients learn how to control their illness themselves, however, they may need mental health visits only once a month. That may not seem like a big deal, but it is. To manage such a devastating diagnosis on one's own for a whole month requires both an acceptance of one's illness and vigilance in taking medications. The client has to believe that they are worthy of care and take good care of themselves on their own, twenty-nine days each month. There's no dollar amount for that.

The holistic approach of the Housing First + ACT model sometimes generates unexpected benefits, which occasionally *do* have a precise dollar value. Rick and a client were watching TV together when a news story upset the client. Here's Rick's summary of the conversation that followed:

> Client: I defended the governor on the steps of the capitol and this is the thanks we get?!
> Rick: You know you're a veteran?
> Client: No.
> Rick: Were you in the military?
> Client: Yeah.
> Rick: Have you ever tried to apply for veterans' benefits?
> Client: No, I don't know what those are.

Rick helped the client apply for his veterans' benefits, which turned out to be almost $100,000. The client became proud to be a veteran. No doubt receiving the money was great, but feeling so highly valued by his country may have been even better. Something like this could only happen because members of the REACT team make time to sit with clients and learn about their lives.

* * *

Housing First is a public policy with a strong evidence base, but it doesn't work for everyone. Many participants fail to keep their housing for the same reasons they were chronically homeless to begin with: substance use disorder, mental health instability, poverty, toxic relationships, and so forth. These people need something different, and not just ineffective short-term detoxification. Detox programs alone fail to outperform untreated withdrawal in preventing relapse. An innovative program in Utah flips the Housing First model by concentrating first on the many root causes of homelessness. Preliminary results are promising.

The Other Side Village is a tiny cottage home community in Salt Lake City for people who have experienced chronic homelessness and struggle with mental health challenges. Eventually, 430 homes are planned, but it is still early days. Around ten people had moved into their homes in May 2025 when I spoke to Moe Egan and Robbie Myrick. Like all the staff, Moe and Robbie have lived experience with homelessness, addiction, mental health, and incarceration. And all of the staff live on the campus. If someone tells Moe they can't do it, Moe is quick to pull out his mugshot from 1999 and says, "Look at this guy, if I can do it, you can do it. And we all have our before and after shots."

Everyone who enters The Other Side Village program is assigned a peer "coach." In the prep program, each coach has only five or six mentees. The ratio goes up to ten mentees per coach after people graduate into their homes. This allows for "very high touch" tailored coaching directed toward "whole-person change," Robbie explained. It could be anything from help getting a GED (high school equivalency degree), to exploring art, to managing difficulty being in crowds. Coaches look for challenging moments to build coping skills little by little and sit with struggling mentees through their darkest hours to inspire hope: Just "make it to your pillow tonight" and "start again tomorrow," as Robbie puts it.

As noted earlier, The Other Side Village does not follow the Housing First model. Placement into the community comes only after a six- to twelve-month prep school, which includes detox and developing the skills and habits needed to be a good member of the community and to hold down a job. Housing is not free. Residents—called "neighbors"—must pay between $250 and $500 each month for rent. Jobs are available at several social enterprises run by The Other Side Village or its sister organization, The Other Side Academy (for criminally involved individuals without mental health challenges). Moe gave this example: "We've got people that were on the streets eight months, a year ago, that now get up at three o'clock in the morning. They make donuts, deliver donuts, and work in our donut shops. It's a human-first issue." With work comes dignity and empowerment. Housing vouchers without life skills don't address the underlying causes of homelessness, Moe explained.

Not everyone makes it through the prep school, but 80 percent have so far. Those who do not were voted out by the other participants and staff, because it is a democratic community. Every person counts equally. The success stories are remarkable. One person with a very low IQ from multiple traumatic brain injuries now works a full-time job and pays his own rent. Another person who had been a patient at a psychiatric facility for eight months without speaking or leaving their room was completely unrecognizable to the staff when they visited the facility again. Notably, with mental health medications, Robbie reports that the problem they see more often is too many meds, rather than too few. There may be medication to sleep and medication to wake up. Sometimes, a new support network can eliminate the need for some medications. A strong community can counteract the "soft bigotry of low expectations," as Moe put it.

I asked Moe if there were any success stories that surprised even him. He told me about the time he "pretty much pulled" a longtime heroin user "off their deathbed" and carried them to a detox program, not knowing "if they're going to make it or not." The program said the person was too sedated, so Moe had to take them to an emergency room first before taking them back to the program. "Four days later they called me and said, 'Moe, what do I do from here?' Just blew me away and I said, 'I'm on my way to pick you up,' so I've learned there's not one person you can write off."

* * *

One question that arises with every housing placement is whether clients should be housed together in one place (the "congregate model") or separately (the "scattered site" model). Rafael's building is an example of the former and the REACT team in Birmingham is an example of the latter. Scattered-site housing can lead to isolation and loneliness. That is the accepted explanation for why the congregate model has generally been found to produce better mental health outcomes.

Avoiding loneliness is no doubt critical, but there's another explanation for the success of the congregate model. Rafael felt it the first time he was housed in a group setting: The residents understand one another ("a bullshitter knows bullshit"). People who have lived through similar challenges connect on a deeper level. The congregate model is effective not only because it reduces loneliness, but also because it unleashes the potential of informal peer support.

The original plan for Rafael's building was to provide only temporary housing while the residents worked on finding permanent housing elsewhere. They quickly discovered a problem with that plan: No one wanted to move out. One of the reasons was that they did not want to lose their sense of community. There is a common space where people gather frequently. At least once a month, there is a community forum where residents have an opportunity to express their concerns. Potlucks include food provided by Rafael's organization, the Wildflower Alliance. And, true to his culinary background, Rafael bought a grill for burgers and hot dogs. This is the "congregate model" working well.

However, plans to house people with mental illness together sometimes run into opposition from the surrounding neighborhood. It's a common enough phenomenon to have a familiar acronym: NIMBY ("Not In My Back Yard"). That wasn't a problem for Rafael's building, but for the wrong reason: The building is in an undesirable neighborhood. Achieving a supportive community within the building may have been possible only by sacrificing the quality of the community immediately outside the building.

Because it adopts the scattered-site model, the REACT program in Birmingham illustrates different complexities and trade-offs. The REACT director, Duncan Gibson, recognizes that integration into the community is the hardest outcome to achieve for many clients: "We're so busy making sure people have their food [and] medicine." Some clients feel lonely and isolated. The COVID pandemic showed that these feelings are grounded in reality. The REACT team was terrified early in the pandemic that, because their clients had so many risk factors, many of them would die of COVID. None did, but also for the wrong reason: "They don't socialize [or go] anywhere."

The scattered-site model mitigates some of the risks of the congregate model. There was a time when the REACT program housed many clients together. The housing coordinator, Rick Gish, told me the story. Years ago, the team had twenty-five clients all in one building. A fire in the building displaced all of them at once, creating a logistical nightmare. Now, "we try not to have all our eggs in one basket," Rick explains. Even smaller numbers of clients housed together can cause serious problems. During Rick's tenure, five clients housed together all relapsed into illegal substance use after one of them did. Even so, Rick never puts one client in an apartment building entirely on their own—there are always at least two clients per building.

But even just two clients living near one another can lead to troublesome disputes, which perhaps isn't surprising since paranoid delusions are a common symptom of schizophrenia and schizoaffective disorder. The congregate model may work better for individuals with less severe diagnoses. In addition, the congregate housing options in Birmingham are terrible. The director of REACT gave this example: A typical boardinghouse has five or six people in one bedroom. She suggested a community of separate tiny homes instead, which is an approach that has worked well elsewhere. In 2023, the City of Birmingham authorized tiny home communities, but that effort has so far been stymied by NIMBY objections.

Scattered-site housing is better than no housing, and it does not have to lead to isolation. To the contrary, having a more permanent place to live makes maintaining social connections easier. While moving into an apartment, one client asked Gish whether he had a cell phone. Televisions and phones are considered "luxuries" and are therefore not covered by the program. The client asked Rick to call the client's mother, whom he had not seen in ten years. The client now had an address to give his mother. She came to visit and has now been a part of the client's life for the last four years.

Two clients in the REACT program go to great lengths, literally, to maintain their friendship. The two friends ended up in apartments across town from each other. Without telling anyone on the team or asking for a ride, one of them walks five miles each way twice a week to visit his friend. It's always the younger and healthier one who makes the trek; the older friend is less mobile. Of course, it would be better if there were appropriate apartments closer together, but their visits are only possible because they are housed and therefore in the same place each week.

Another story from the REACT team illustrates the strength of the community that can form among people who are unhoused. Sometimes, when there are no appropriate one-bedroom apartments available, Rick can get approval for a two-bedroom apartment. He doesn't do that very often anymore for a reason you might not expect. More than once, the day after moving a client into a two-bedroom apartment, Rick will return to find additional people staying there. "Why are they here?" "Well, 'cause they were homeless, too. I'm just trying to pay it forward." Rick reluctantly has to explain that the program doesn't allow any roommates.

* * *

The REACT team has eighteen multidisciplinary members to serve 103 patients, including a full-time peer. In contrast, Rafael works ten to fifteen hours each week as the only peer in a building with forty-six single-occupancy rooms. Of course, with this staff-to-client ratio, Rafael cannot match the time, intensity, or variety of supports offered by the REACT team. Still, Rafael told me repeatedly that he provides "wraparound" services. Skeptical, I eventually asked him directly what he meant by "wraparound." Are there any employment supports or educational programs?

Rafael looked at me a little funny before explaining that his version of wraparound supports includes "anything that you can conceive, we can strive together to look for it." No goal is too lofty. He gave this example:

> *I wanna move to the lower East Side and have a penthouse in the sky. . . . I'm not there to do stuff for people. I will support you to learn to do it for yourself. That way, when it happens in the future, you know what to do. And so that's the real goal. . . . It doesn't necessarily have to do with moving towards something, but just overall, you know, fulfilling something within your life.*

Rafael really does just about "anything" for the residents of Greenville. When he first started working there, an older female resident said directly what many other residents were probably thinking: "I don't know about you. I don't trust you." She later occasionally said "some pretty awful, racist stuff." But the woman eventually came around and referred to Rafael as her "Puerto Rican angel." Their relationship became so close that when the woman was sick in the hospital, her daughter called Rafael and said, "Hey, I think my mom would really want you to be here and say goodbye." "And so," Rafael concluded, "I was able to do that."

TAKEAWAYS

- A safe and stable place to stay can be essential to living successfully with mental illness.
- There are evidence-based programs, like Housing First, to improve housing and related outcomes.

- Some people will prefer group housing, others will prefer tiny home communities, and many need help overcoming substance use disorders.
- Peers are helping each other find and maintain quality housing and build more meaningful lives.

CHAPTER 7

EMPLOYMENT

"I'm pretty resilient."

Samantha Smith is a master of understatement. Her mental health struggles began early. Samantha suffered abuse and trauma at home as a child. By age eight, she had begun thinking about suicide and even talked about it at school. The school counselor called her in, but offered no support. The effect was shame and ridicule from other students. She doesn't know whether anyone at the school told her family, but the subject was never discussed at home.

Samantha continued to struggle, but a decade would pass before she received any mental health treatment. Shortly after starting college, she was diagnosed with chronic depression and generalized anxiety disorder. She found counseling helpful, but she stopped when she graduated—she wanted "to just do life on [her] own." Samantha thought she was doing fine, and she was, until a breakup in 2017 sent her on a new downward spiral. Unable to keep a job, Samantha briefly went on short-term disability. Samantha attempted suicide multiple times, beginning in college and continuing until as recently as 2019.

When I spoke to her in 2023, Samantha was the executive administrator for operations at a large Dallas-area church. Working at the church allowed Samantha to advance her mission to help other people. Researching and embracing religion were keys to her own recovery. "You have to understand the science of what you're going through, and you have to understand it from your spiritual perspective of how that fits into your purpose, your world, everything like that." The moment she drew this connection, Samantha's suicidal thoughts "went away" and her depression "kind of got cured." Now, depressive thoughts represent an attack from an external enemy; those thoughts do not reflect her true self.

Samantha lived long enough to reach that moment of epiphany only through more traditional mental healthcare. She found the community and support of group therapy to be extremely helpful. Telling and hearing each other's stories reduced Samantha's feelings of isolation. During the COVID-19 pandemic, a particularly astute therapist helped Samantha uncover her own positive mindset: "If you were hopeless or you really wanted to die, you wouldn't log into these meetings like you do; you wouldn't be doing the work that you're doing."

Samantha knows she is lucky. She is grateful for having survived without being admitted to a hospital, even during suicidal periods so severe that she probably needed twenty-four-hour monitoring. Samantha avoided not just involuntary hospitalization, but involuntary treatment of any kind. As we've seen, experiencing forced treatment drives many away from the mental healthcare system (recall Jesse Mangan from chapter 2). Even after her moment of insight and the stability she has enjoyed since, Samantha does not reject science-based mental healthcare. She takes pride in being able to stay healthy without medication, but she recognizes that medications may be needed in times of crisis.

Samantha is quite happy with the mental healthcare she received: "I have actually never run into, like, a bad experience in my mental journey with hospitals . . . I've always had amazing therapists . . . [they were] awesome to me." Why was Samantha's experience so much less coercive and so much more effective than almost everyone else's in this book?

There are many reasons, of course, but perhaps the single biggest reason was private health insurance. Amazingly, even during her deep and recurring depressive episodes, Samantha remained fully employed, except for one small stint on short-term disability. Each job provided her with health insurance. We've seen that our mental healthcare "system" is fractured into many different systems: crisis, criminal, inpatient, outpatient, and so on. Samantha's experience underscores another gaping divide between private and public mental healthcare systems.

Between 2017 and 2020, Samantha participated in three Intensive Outpatient Programs (IOPs), which ranged in duration from one to four months depending on the severity of the depressive episode. Before each IOP, Samantha started in "partial hospitalization," which consists of in-person programming from 8:00 a.m. to 5:00 p.m. every weekday. Patients spend the entire workweek at the hospital but get to go home each night. Patients who do well typically "step down" to an IOP, which includes fewer and shorter in-person sessions. Intensive programs like these are expensive, too expensive to be included in public benefits programs. Samantha did her IOPs at one of the top three psychiatric hospitals in Dallas. "I had jobs where I had great insurance. I could never have done three IOP programs without my work, without my jobs, ever. That would not have ever happened." In other words, Samantha survived only because she had the almost unbelievable tenacity to show up every day for her full-time job and perform well enough to keep it during suicidal episodes so extreme that many would think the hospital would have been the only safe place for her.

There are very few people with that kind of strength. Many other mental health conditions have symptoms that cannot be concealed and may make it impossible to work during acute episodes. People with those conditions are unlikely to be able to keep a full-time job with benefits. Some don't bother to apply for jobs; others later get fired. Underemployment or unemployment, in turn, means no access to lifesaving, or substantially life-improving, treatments that only private health insurance will cover. People who need quality mental healthcare to be able to work are denied that care precisely because they are unable to work without having it. Private health insurance is reserved for the people who need it least. Samantha is an exception that proves the rule. She was able to access the intensive treatment that saved her life only because she miraculously kept her job during periods when she had no business being anywhere outside of a hospital.

Samantha's advocacy work began early and has continued unabated through her own periods of crisis. She joined the Texas Protection and Advocacy for Individuals with Mental Illness Advisory Council in 2017. When we spoke in 2023, she was also on the board of Disability

Rights Texas. She has directly lobbied state legislators. Outside of Texas, Samantha has become a nationally recognized advocate for mental health reform. She is on the board of the National Association for Rights Protection and Advocacy. Samantha has worked with other national organizations, including Mental Health America and National Alliance on Mental Illness. And she is certified in one-on-one suicide intervention.

"Pretty resilient," indeed.

* * *

Quality mental healthcare through employer-provided insurance has benefits in every aspect of life for someone with a mental illness. Stable mental health makes everything else easier. But a job means so much more than health insurance.

People with serious mental illnesses want to work a job for the same reasons as everyone else: achieving economic stability and having a sense of purpose. But employment is even more meaningful to a person with SMI. A job represents a step back into society, toward dignity and self-worth. Stephanie Nieves, the employment program director at Fountain House, explains:

> *Seeing people get their first paycheck, and how excited they are, like their first-ever paycheck is something really emotional, I think. That still moves me, after all of these years, to see how excited people are about, like, "I did it." . . .*
>
> *I think what we see a lot in the desire to work a lot from folks at Fountain House is a desire for normalcy. For "See, I'm just like everybody else. I'm working. I can do it." That, I think, is the motivator for a lot of folks.*

This is not unique to Fountain House. Most people receiving treatment for SMI list employment as one of their most important goals, and the benefits are well-established.

Consistent with Stephanie's experience, research shows that employment improves self-esteem, quality of life, social relationships, and community integration. The positive personal and social effects of employment are probably not surprising. What may be surprising is that having a job also reduces psychiatric symptoms, psychiatric hospitalizations, and overall mental health spending. Employment interventions have been shown to be effective and relatively inexpensive. These findings led two researchers in 2020 to argue that "helping people with employment should be a standard mental health intervention."

The employment figures for people with SMI are abysmal. Estimates of the unemployment rate range from 55 percent to 82 percent. A 2008 study calculated that these lost earnings cost society $193.2 billion annually. The lost benefits to individuals with SMI is much higher than that. The Fountain House members Stephanie works with are overjoyed with their first paychecks not because of the amount, but because of what the paycheck represents. Being a full participant in society is what matters most. That feeling, and the work itself, lead to clinical improvement. The notion that work is central to human flourishing dates back to antiquity, but studies dating back to the 1980s have suggested that work improves "even the most basic symptoms of severe mental illness such as schizophrenia." Many potential gains are lost when so many people are unemployed.

* * *

There are many reasons why the employment rate among people with mental illness is so tragically low. They face unique challenges at every step of the process. As a result, they are less likely to apply, less likely to be hired, and more likely to be fired. Some of the hurdles are obvious, but some are not.

Good intentions can lead to bad results. Public benefits programs are designed to help those who need it most, which makes perfect sense given budget constraints. It is also reasonable for the government to believe that a person with significant employment income is less needy than people without a job. When income exceeds the threshold, a person can lose their benefits. That's okay for people like Samantha who can secure and keep good-paying jobs with generous private health insurance. Not everyone has those skills, fortitude, and good fortune.

By penalizing work, public benefits programs create a trap. Many jobs available to people with mental illness do not provide health insurance or other benefits. A person who is receiving public benefits—including mental healthcare—can lose those crucial benefits if they have a paying job too long and earn above a certain threshold. The income threshold is quite low: Anything more than a part-time job at minimum wage can be disqualifying. Working more hours or working at a higher pay rate can create a net financial loss. Christina Fox, a peer employment specialist, explains: "They come out making less money from working than what they would have received before."

Losing a job with benefits can be catastrophic for people with substantial mental healthcare needs. Restarting benefits is a slow, difficult process. In the meantime, the person may not have sufficient resources to meet even their most basic needs. Finding a replacement job in such dire circumstances may not be realistic. Working is like walking a tightrope without a net. Many people who want to work, and who could work successfully, rationally decide not to take the risk. And some of the brave souls who risk employment will not succeed and will be left without even basic life necessities.

Recent policy changes have improved the situation, but the programs are still complicated, and the fear remains. Tammy Melvin is herself a peer specialist focused on employment (at Jefferson Blount St. Clair Mental Health Authority), but she still lives with this uncertainty:

> *The possibility [of losing benefits] scares me to death. . . . Part-time work would not afford me to live, so I'm just trusting God. Really . . . it's just one of those things that I don't understand. I really don't. I've heard so many different things from, you know . . . Social Security and benefits counselors, so like I said, I'm just, you know, trusting God that that will work itself out.*

Even though the risk of losing your job and your benefits never goes away, many public employment assistance programs are limited to six or nine months, Tammy explained. At JBS, though, the peers are allowed to stay in contact with clients even after the case has been formally closed. That's why JBS peer Marie Holliday was able to reopen a case to help a former client who was "really stressed out" at work. Marie's first question was: "What are you doing to take care of yourself?" "Nothing," the woman answered; she was too busy working. "Well, on your off days, don't answer the phone," Marie advised. The woman was incredulous; she thought she had to answer, especially as a supervisor. The woman decided to look for another job. Marie officially reopened the case, and the woman landed a better job. Later, the woman called to tell Marie that she got nominated to be employee of the month. "That is fantastic. You know, you're where they appreciate the hard work that you do." Support for as long as needed is critical to keep people employed and to find them better positions. And knowing that support will always be there may even be enough to convince some individuals to take the big first step of looking for a job.

* * *

Fear of losing benefits is not the only reason that people with mental illness decide not to apply for a job. Another reason is the belief that, because of their illness, they cannot do the job. For some people that may be true, but not for many others. People with serious mental illness are often capable of more than they realize.

One evidence-based employment intervention for individuals with mental illness is the Individual Placement and Support model of Supported Employment (IPS or IPS+SE). Importantly, the model is open to anyone who wants to work—regardless of diagnosis, symptoms, housing status, or most anything else. Counselors explain the potential effects on benefits up front. The goal of IPS is generally a regular paid position open to people without mental illness—in other words, a "competitive" position—not a volunteer or segregated position, because competitive employment is what most people want. People are placed into jobs as quickly as possible, without extensive training, then provided with indefinite long-term support. The commitment to rapid placement distinguishes IPS from traditional train-first-place-later vocational rehabilitation models.

The outcomes achieved by IPS may be surprising. One might predict that rushing even the most disabled clients into competitive employment with little or no training would be disastrous. The opposite is true. A 2023 analysis of scores of randomized controlled trials (RCTs) concluded that IPS increases the rate of competitive employment by about twice as much as other models. Outcomes are *worse* for programs that provide preplacement training than for models that prioritize rapid placement. And by skipping expensive testing and training, IPS achieves these better outcomes at a lower cost. The core premise of IPS is that everyone with SMI can obtain and keep a paid job. It's hard to argue with the results.

People with lived experience are already helping one another find and keep jobs in many different ways, formal and informal. Fountain House prioritizes celebrating members' employment successes. Members talk about their experiences and encourage others to do it: "I did do this job. I did it well, you should do it too, you would like it," Stephanie recounts. At the formal end of the spectrum, research shows that peers can be trained to provide IPS services effectively.

* * *

Even if a person with SMI believes in their own abilities, they may choose not to apply for a job because they are afraid of being discriminated against by employers and coworkers. This fear is so common that it has a name: "anticipated discrimination." And while the fear of discrimination may sometimes be worse than the reality, there is no doubt that employment discrimination is real. It's also illegal, sort of.

In the landmark *Wyatt* case (see chapter 2), Judge Johnson recognized for the first time a federal constitutional right to treatment in state psychiatric facilities. Understaffing at Alabama's Bryce Hospital made it impossible for the facility to provide adequate care, so Judge Johnson ordered the hospital to maintain minimum staff-to-patient ratios. Jon Brock took advantage of the opportunity and applied for a job. He sat across a desk from the woman conducting the interview. She opened his application and asked, "Why do you want to work at Bryce?"

> *"Naturally," I replied, "Well, I used to be a patient here and . . ." I never finished since she folded my application, moved it to the side of her desk, nearest the garbage can I noticed, and then said, "We don't hire people at Bryce who have been patients here." Bryce Hospital had been there well over a century at that point and . . . counted people who had been through their care and treatment as entities . . . not to be trusted, not to be thought of as capable or responsible.*

Jon has told me this story more than once. It is both disturbing and revealing, and not just about attitudes toward former patients of Bryce. Discrimination against people with mental illness would not be declared illegal until almost two decades later. The woman knew she did not have to hide her reason for rejecting Jon's application.

The federal Americans with Disabilities Act of 1990 (ADA) prohibits employers from discriminating against people because of their "mental disabilities." That term includes mental health diagnoses if the condition "substantially limits one or more major life activities." Examples of such activities include "walking," "talking," "performing manual tasks," and "working." That means an employer cannot refuse to hire, or choose to fire, people with certain conditions that seriously limit their ability to work. Does that mean employers must hire and retain employees who cannot do the job? No.

The ADA, unlike other civil rights laws, requires employers to provide "reasonable accommodations" to disabled employees. In other words, employers may be required to modify job duties or work environments if the modifications will allow a disabled employee to do a job that they wouldn't otherwise be able to do. A simple example of a "reasonable accommodation" for a physical disability is building a ramp that allows a person in a wheelchair to get to their desk. On the other hand, the same employer would not be required to put in an expensive elevator if it were deemed an "undue hardship."

A person in a wheelchair will have a hard time concealing their condition during an in-person job interview. In contrast, most mental disabilities can be hidden. To make unlawful discrimination more difficult, employers are prohibited from asking about disabilities before they make a job offer. Nor may employers use any criterion that appears neutral but has a disparate negative impact on people with disabilities. After making an offer, employers can ask about disabilities that impact "essential job functions" and determine whether the applicant can perform these functions, either with or without reasonable accommodations.

Of course, not every person with a disability will be able to perform the essential functions of every job, even with all the modifications required by the ADA. An employer is not obligated to hire such a person and not prohibited from firing that person later. For example, an airline can refuse to hire someone as a pilot if they have uncontrolled epilepsy or terrible vision. Some people with serious mental illness are unable to do some jobs, either due to symptoms or due to the side effects of medications. Finding a job that they can do without accommodation is the main hurdle for many people with SMI, as the overall success of IPS demonstrates. But IPS does not work for everyone: Some folks need more help.

* * *

Stephanie Nieves has a master's degree in community psychology. She has worked at Fountain House for about ten years, the last four on the employment team, including the last two or three as its director. "The community is based on work." Every member is encouraged to engage in structured activities that contribute to the community. This is called the "work-ordered day." Stephanie explains that the goal is to give members a feeling of purpose by working each day for the benefit of the community. The work could happen anywhere from the garden to the kitchen to the art gallery.

Fountain House and the many clubhouses around the world inspired by it are examples of peers helping each other. Many members will not look for employment outside the clubhouse. Some have never applied for jobs on their own, or have not done so for a very long time. Others do not want another job, or have pronounced symptoms, including "active hallucinations and delusions," which can be difficult to manage in competitive workplaces. On the other hand, Stephanie is quick to point out that "we have a lot of people who do work independently and have for years with very little support."

A member who wants to work outside of Fountain House, but needs some help to do so, has several options. Transitional employment (TE) positions are reserved for members at independent firms or organizations. Fountain House assumes responsibility for the job functions and fills TE positions with members it believes can succeed. Placement is only the first step. Fountain House continues to provide individualized support throughout the TE position, hopefully with declining levels of intensity as the member becomes more comfortable in the position.

These TE positions are all part-time, entry-level, and pay at market rates. They are intended to last six to nine months, though this time limit can be waived. For example, Cyrus Napolitano's (chapter 5) TE position scanning documents at a large, international law firm lasted eight years. The firm was happy with Cyrus's work and Cyrus was happy with the job. It was with obvious pride that Cyrus told me that the extended time period allowed him to finish the massive scanning job that was his primary assignment at the firm. Transitional employment can provide members who want permanent employment with a safe and supported way to learn by doing.

Critically, the TE program is designed so that participants do not risk losing government benefits. Participants are paid a fair wage, but their hours are limited so as not to disqualify them from benefits programs. Higher take-home pay for longer periods of time can disqualify participants from receiving disability benefits, even though their new income may not be sufficient to cover basic needs. The skills needed for a particular TE position are often less important than lessons like punctuality and professionalism. Based on the member's experiences during the TE, they will be much better able to decide whether to try for a permanent position, either below or above the income level that could lead to a loss of benefits. Fountain House guides them through that complicated and high-stakes decision-making process.

Sometimes, transitional employment gives members the opportunity to develop unexpected skills, which can be life-changing even if the member never works again. With obvious delight, Stephanie told me the story of one "very funny" member, Leon.* Leon's first TE position

---

* Not his real name.

was supposed to be in an office. He was so excited that he showed up way too early. That happens a lot, Stephanie explained. Showing up too early on the first day of TE is much more common than showing up late. Members are usually eager to get to work. When Leon's new supervisors finally arrived at the office, they found him gesturing expansively and "interacting . . . with something that [was] obviously not clear to everybody around him." Note the language Stephanie uses. Leon saw something that others could not. A doctor would call this a "hallucination," but for Leon it was real. Leon was so excited that he even danced a little. The supervisors complained to Fountain House, and Leon was unable to start the position. Leon was saddened, but that's not the end of his story.

The next TE position that Fountain House found for Leon was food delivery to individuals with mobility challenges, "basically delivering meals on wheels on foot." In this job, no one would notice (or care) if Leon sometimes acted in a manner that would be inappropriate in an office. But Leon had to overcome a different hurdle: The deliveries were in tall buildings in New York City. "I don't do elevators," Leon declared. With encouragement, Leon decided to accept the position. In the end, his fear of elevators was not as strong as his desire to work.

Fountain House provided more than just encouragement. "You can do it" and "you want to work" were followed up with *"we're* gonna do this." Stephanie trained Leon on one of his first days. "I remember we would have to just push every button in the elevator . . . one on every floor, so that it wouldn't drop too quickly." Leon may not have made many friends among the other riders of that busy elevator, but he confronted and overcame his fear. It wasn't long before he stopped pushing every button. This may seem like a small victory, but it wasn't. When you live in New York City, being able to ride an elevator is a very big deal. A huge portion of the city is located on floors higher than anyone would want to have to reach by climbing stairs. Elevators don't open every door, but they can at least put you in a position to knock on them.

* * *

Over 90 percent of U.S. employers check applicants for a criminal record. Applicants will usually learn this from the job posting or the application. Most people with a criminal record simply won't apply, the few that do apply will likely be rejected, and essentially none will be able to afford a legal challenge. Requiring a clean record sounds reasonable and is neutral on its face, but it disqualifies a disproportionate share of individuals with substance use and other mental health disorders. Subject to a few exceptions, the ADA is supposed to prohibit employment practices that have this kind of disparate impact on people with disabilities, even when the employer does not intend to discriminate. It may be possible to have criminal convictions expunged, but that process can be expensive, and it is not available in some states for common offenses like assault and domestic violence. Much better to avoid getting a criminal record in the first place. Mental health courts (described in chapter 3) provide that opportunity. Treatment rather than punishment is the goal for people whose illness caused their misconduct.

* * *

The ADA prohibits employment discrimination based on mental as well as physical disabilities. There are no blood tests to diagnose mental illness. Diagnoses are based primarily on observed and self-reported behaviors. Indeed, the term "behavioral health" is sometimes used as a synonym of "mental health." Under the ADA, it is illegal to fire an employee merely for having a qualifying mental health diagnosis. However, that can change quickly when the first symptom appears.

The United States is divided into twelve geographic federal courts of appeals, which sometimes reach different conclusions on legal questions. In most of the country, "If an employer fires an employee because of the employee's unacceptable behavior, the fact that that behavior was precipitated by a mental illness does not present an issue under the Americans with Disabilities Act." That "majority rule" means employers can avoid the ADA altogether simply by classifying annoying behavioral symptoms of mental illness as "unacceptable." A mental disability is literally defined by behavior, but behaviors caused by the disability are not protected.* Does the ADA protect only people without symptoms? Does a person without symptoms even have a disability or need protection against discrimination?

A few federal appeals courts follow a "minority rule" instead. These courts recognize that "if the law fails to protect the manifestations of [a] disability, there is no real protection in the law because it would protect the disabled in name only." As a result, employers will sometimes be required to "tolerate eccentric or unusual conduct" by employees who can still perform the essential functions of their jobs. Put another way, employers remain free to discipline or terminate employees for a behavior caused by a disability if the behavior violates a conduct rule that is "job-related for the position in question and consistent with business necessity."

An example from the Equal Employment Opportunity Commission shows what's at stake in choosing between these two approaches. Suppose an employee loads boxes all day in a warehouse. He has no regular contact with other employees, and he has no contact at all with customers. What he does have is schizophrenia. The illness never affects his job performance, but during occasional acute phases, the employee becomes disheveled and rude. The company terminates him for violating its policies that require every employee to maintain "a neat appearance" and to be "courteous" at all times.

Under the majority rule, the employer has not violated the ADA. Being "disheveled" and "rude" in the workplace is "unacceptable." So long as the company enforces its rules even-handedly, there is no violation. The fact that the violations were caused by a mental disability does not matter to most federal appellate courts. That is not true under the minority view: An employer cannot take adverse action against an employee for misconduct caused by a disability, unless the relevant

---

* This was the law in Chicago when my two manic episodes, and slow recovery from each, kept me out of the office for several months. Absenteeism surely qualifies as "unacceptable behavior," so my law firm could have legally fired me under this logic. Thankfully, that is not the culture of the firm. Indeed, it was a former named partner of the firm, Judge Milton Shadur, who wrote the more enlightened opinion quoted in the next paragraph.

conduct rule is related to the employee's position and is a "business necessity." Because our hypothetical employee works alone, these two conduct rules are not related to his position. It would be difficult for the employer to show a "business necessity" because the employee's conduct apparently does not affect either productivity or safety. The employer is just going to have to put up with a little rudeness and an unkempt appearance if those idiosyncrasies are caused by a disability.

The bottom line is that an employee with a mental illness should probably hide it completely because their employer may be able to lawfully discriminate against them as soon as the first troublesome symptom appears.

* * *

An employee's decision to tell their employer about their mental health diagnosis is complicated and very high stakes. Beyond the loss of privacy, disclosing the diagnosis opens them up to stigma and discrimination. Of course, discrimination is illegal under the ADA but, as we have just seen, employers are generally allowed to enforce conduct rules even if they know a violation was caused by a mental disability. Disclosure will not help the employee in that circumstance.

There are, however, significant advantages to disclosure. The employer may be sympathetic and provide the employee with helpful support. If the employee wants to request a "reasonable accommodation," then the employee must disclose the disability that needs to be accommodated. People want to be honest; concealment is stressful. Keeping such a big secret requires distancing oneself from coworkers, which hurts job performance and satisfaction. As peer advocate Jon Brock observed, "You find yourself being careful about what you say to who, and then you get more and more isolated, and then after a while, you know, well, that's not working and you're looking for work again." In his vocational rehabilitation efforts, Jon's next move was to find nonprofits willing to hire people knowing that the person had a mental illness. Fountain House uses the same strategy.

But perhaps the most important reason to disclose a diagnosis is that it allows employees to be their true selves: "Authenticity has been shown to be positively related to work engagement, job satisfaction and work performance." The underlying study that reached this conclusion involved Dutch bankers with mental illness; the positive effects would almost certainly be larger for people working in healthcare. And for peer providers and advocates, authenticity is absolutely essential.

Rafael Rodriguez, a peer focused on housing (see chapter 6), explains:

> *I work for an organization [the Wildflower Alliance in Massachusetts] that truly honors my lived experience. So first and foremost, that's number one, right? That I can bring my full authentic self to my work, and it is honored and actually appreciated. And it's not looked down upon or stigmatized. It's actually reinforced and supported. And so that's extremely important to the work that I do.*

Lived experience, and openness about it, are precisely what makes peers effective.

The value of peers in mental healthcare is being recognized more and more. Grants often require peer team members; agencies do the same or have specialized peer divisions. It is no exaggeration to call peer work a "movement." But peers face special challenges working in the mental health sphere. Interactions and stress can be triggering. Too much empathy can lead to burnout or even to crisis.

Melissa Wettengel has thought deeply about the issue of peer workforce sustainability. Early in her life, she had to withdraw from Cornell University after one semester, was hospitalized, and received a diagnosis of manic-depression. Her family was told that she would never be able to go back to school, get married, or have a house, and would probably be in and out of the hospital for the rest of her life. Her mother, a nurse, was having none of that. It took years of struggle, but Melissa eventually proved her mom right and the hospital wrong by achieving all these things and more.

Melissa is now the chief executive officer of Hands Across Long Island, a sixty-person peer services organization. She recognizes that people with mental health challenges often need special support to succeed as peer service providers. Some organizations require peers to meet with clinicians, a strategy that Melissa describes as "actually really dangerous" and "discrimination." Her prescription looks different: "What we found that ultimately supports the workforce and sustains the workforce is having peers work alongside other peers." This is necessarily the case in a purely peer-staffed organization like her own, but the principle can be extrapolated. If peers are spread out in different divisions of an agency, or in different organizations, she recommends setting up a "community of practice," where peers can come together from across agencies to support one another. Melissa created one such community on Long Island when she was in a prior position: "It was about increasing our skills, making sure everyone knew where the trainings were and the conferences, some mentoring we could give each other. Some of it was just mutual support and socializing."

Peers also struggle with respect, role clarity, compensation, and career advancement. Peers are very often supervised by non-peers who do not understand the proper role of a peer. With ill-defined or undefined expectations, peer positions on a team may devolve into tokenism. Opportunities for promotion may be nonexistent. There is an active debate about whether peers should be required to obtain higher degrees. The thinking is that degrees may confer skills but also support claims for better pay and supervisory roles. For example, Melissa went back to school for both her undergraduate degree and a master's degree in public health. "That's just the reality that with initials after our name, we're taken more seriously. And it's a big challenge for our workforce to not be taken seriously."

We do not even know how many working peers there are because the federal government isn't counting. The U.S. Department of Labor does not have an occupational code for peer support specialists, so there are no national statistics. The Providing Empathetic and Effective Recovery Support Act (PEER Support Act) would correct that omission. But even this first small step toward recognition and respect seems very unlikely in the near term after Donald Trump regained the White House and the Republicans took control of Congress in 2025. In the meantime, peers will continue to work in support of one another without the protection and support they deserve from the rest of us.

TAKEAWAYS

- Quality private healthcare is generally accessible only for people well enough to attain and keep a good job.

- People with mental illnesses too serious to stay employed are relegated to generally inferior public healthcare systems.

- Employment is not just the key to better mental healthcare and a living wage—it is key to intangible benefits like increased self-esteem.

- There are well-established, evidence-based interventions that improve employment outcomes for people with serious mental illness.

CHAPTER 8

EDUCATION

Shannon Pagdon still hears voices. She started hearing them in high school, but her struggles in school started much earlier. At age twelve, she was diagnosed with ADHD. Things got worse at sixteen when her nightmares turned into paranoid delusions and visual hallucinations. She eventually couldn't tell whether she was awake or dreaming. It was a nightmare either way. She saw a therapist and a psychiatrist, and was put on "many, many, many different medications." The voices only grew stronger.

Shannon considers the fact that she was able to finish high school "mildly miraculous." She was scaring people by talking to herself in class, so the school sent her home and brought the assignments to her. Shannon thinks now that it was probably "the best that they could offer." Being pulled out of school exacerbated the isolation she felt; friends she had been close to since kindergarten just disappeared. Shannon recognizes that some of her behavior hurt people, but she believes fear of and negative perceptions about psychosis and schizophrenia played a big role. College did not go well. She tried hard for years at different schools, but she "inevitably would get very stressed and then have to withdraw."

Stress wasn't the only problem. Shannon also ran into structural financial barriers. Because of her symptoms, Shannon could attend school only part-time. Because she was part-time, she couldn't qualify for financial aid. The theory, she supposes, is that a part-time student could work and therefore pay their own tuition. That may make sense for people without disabilities, but in effect, it discriminates against people with disabilities. When Shannon once sought disability benefits, she was rejected because she applied under the wrong Social Security program.

Without a college degree, Shannon's work options were limited. She tried many different low-wage jobs. She worked in an ice cream shop and as a barista in a bookstore café. The higher stress levels in jobs like these exacerbated Shannon's symptoms. She didn't tell her employers about her diagnosis because she was afraid of stigma. Instead, when the stress became overwhelming, she would simply quit and look for another job. This cycle continued until she finally landed a position as a peer specialist. She describes the job with words like "reciprocity," "meaningful," "beautiful," and "powerful." Why did she end up quitting the job she loved? It didn't pay enough to cover her expenses.

* * *

People with mental illness want to attend college for the same reasons as everyone else: Some want to learn for learning's sake, and nearly everyone wants to get better jobs. Focusing solely on wages, higher education in the United States is a great investment. In the United States, earning a bachelor's degree increases a person's lifetime income by roughly $1,200,000, as compared to a person with only a high school diploma. A graduate degree adds another $600,000 or so.

People with mental illness benefit from college in other important ways. "Education helped me to find a sense of purpose and transition into other life roles," one graduate explained. Higher education helps people with mental illnesses form identities that go beyond their diagnoses. Each instantly becomes a "student" and in turn can become an aspiring "lawyer," "doctor," "engineer," or "professor." Education has benefits in other domains as well. For example, a study of the clubhouse model created at Fountain House found that educational attainment was associated with greater perceived effectiveness in a wide variety of social settings. Research has also identified improvements in self-confidence and self-concept.

Notwithstanding all these benefits, higher education is out of reach for many individuals with mental illness. They are much less likely to complete college or graduate school. One 2005 study estimated that 86 percent of college students with serious mental illness drop out. That's way higher than the overall dropout rate. Similar disparities exist in high school as well, so there are fewer qualified college applicants with mental illness. Young adulthood is the peak of mental illness onset. In addition to the shock caused by the diagnosis, the new symptoms may take a long time to get under control. At the same time, going to college often decreases support from family and friends and increases loneliness and financial strain.

The illness itself makes college harder. Common symptoms of mental illness, like reduced stamina and trouble focusing, can significantly impair a college student's performance. But sometimes the cure is worse than the disease. The side effects of even the most effective psychiatric medications can be disabling in other ways. For example, one of Shannon's antipsychotic medications made her hands shake so badly that she couldn't read her own writing. Thankfully, the school provided her with a notetaker.*

Since 1990, the ADA has required colleges to make "reasonable accommodations" like providing a notetaker. Another common example is providing a separate examination room for a student who has difficulty screening out environmental distractions. Of course, accommodations don't just happen. Colleges have to know about a disability in order to accommodate it. Research shows that about half of university students experiencing mental health problems do not seek professional help. Students may be reluctant to disclose their diagnosis for a variety of good reasons, and many students are not aware that they are entitled to accommodations. Even those who disclose and request an accommodation may have to wait a long time to receive it.

***

---

* What comes around sometimes goes around. Diagnosed with bipolar disorder, jailed, and hospitalized three times for psychosis, Eric Smith (chapter 4) went on to become a notetaker for another student with a disability.

Doing a better job addressing these challenges in higher education would obviously have huge benefits for students with mental illness. Ignore the massive individual benefits for the moment. Less obviously, evidence-based interventions produce huge public benefits as well. As previously discussed, higher educational attainment is associated with higher income. People with higher incomes don't qualify for a range of government benefits, hopefully because they don't need them (but see chapter 7). Those disability benefits are very expensive and are ultimately paid for by taxpayers. In this way, improving the education outcomes—and by extension, increasing the incomes—of people with mental illness can benefit all of us.

But this positive effect happens only if interventions to improve educational outcomes actually reduce disability benefits by more than the cost of the interventions themselves. A 2019 study examined whether this was the case for an experimental two-year intervention called Recovery After an Initial Schizophrenia Episode Early Treatment Program (RAISE-ETP). RAISE-ETP included collaborative medical management, family psychoeducation, and educational or employment support. Providing this type of holistic care was not cheap.

The study estimated that it would cost $4.2 billion to scale up the program to include every eligible person. On the other side of the ledger, national implementation would result in an estimated reduction in disability expenditures of—wait for it—$8.9 billion. That's an outstanding return on investment. The cost of expanding this program to help young people with schizophrenia would pay for itself more than twice over. Even if taxpayers care nothing about people with a mental illness and just want to lower taxes, they should be demanding evidence-based educational programs like RAISE-ETP. And, again, we aren't even including benefits to the individual participants. The same study estimated increased lifetime earnings of 7 percent ($40,900). Other research shows that the RAISE-ETP program reduced clinical symptoms, improved social and occupational functioning, and increased school and work participation.

Other models of coordinated specialty care—the generic term for programs like RAISE-ETP—also produce positive effects. Comprehensive and better coordinated services are critical, but so is the shift to a more person-centered approach. Participants describe staff as taking their opinions seriously and expressing "no judgment at all." People with lived experience of psychosis are uniquely qualified to connect with other people dealing with this profoundly destabilizing experience for the first time.

RAISE-ETP is not a panacea. The program is for first-episode psychosis only, so even if fully implemented, it would benefit only a small percentage of people with mental illness. Interventions for other mental health symptoms may or may not pay for themselves in disability benefits saved, but this one fiscal benefit barely scratches the surface of even purely economic gains, like increased income tax revenue and lower public spending on healthcare. Other types of benefits like improved quality of life, social effectiveness, and self-worth are impossible to quantify. The most important policy lessons of the RAISE-ETP project are to incorporate non-pharmacological interventions and to adopt a broader view of the relevant costs and benefits.

* * *

Shannon was living in New York City when she heard about Fountain House (see chapter 5). Fountain House operates the nation's largest Supported Education (SEd) program for people with mental illness. Details vary, but SEd programs help participants set educational goals, build academic skills, and improve motivation, both in one-on-one interactions with specialized staff and in group workshops. SEd programs also facilitate enrollment, assist in obtaining financial aid and accommodations, and connect participants to mental health and other needed services. SEd is not a segregated training program; participants attend the same schools and classes as students without disabilities.

Shannon walked through the door as a "self-referral" and quickly connected with the college reentry program. That was the first semester she completed any college classes. The reentry program at Fountain House recognizes that success in college requires more than just academic skills. There are classes on personal finance and cooking. In

Shannon's view, "things like that are such important aspects of life that are completely left out of a more clinical focus program and early intervention program."

When asked what aspects of the program worked for her, Shannon responded without hesitation: "The most powerful thing was peer support." It was the first time she had talked to another person with "any kind of lived experience of a nonconsensus reality." Fountain House assigned Shannon a one-on-one mentor who also had experience with psychosis. "We would go out and get a cup of coffee and talk, and it was so normalizing and lovely to connect." Clubhouses can become a new family. Shannon "celebrated [her] twenty-first birthday at the Fountain House farm." Getting back into college was just the beginning for Shannon. Like many SEd participants, she set and achieved the higher goal of earning a bachelor's degree.

* * *

In 2015, a twenty-year-old Yale student named Luchang Wang was struggling with mental health problems. She explained in a Facebook post that she "couldn't bear the thought of leaving school for a full year, or of leaving and never being readmitted." Instead of withdrawing from Yale, Luchang flew to San Francisco and jumped to her death off the Golden Gate Bridge. In response, Yale made a few changes to its readmission policy, but students still feared seeking treatment on campus or taking time off to recover.

The tragedy was repeated six years later. First-year student Rachael Shaw-Rosenbaum was a talented violist with a passion for justice. Her dream was to become a Supreme Court justice like her hero, Ruth Bader Ginsburg. Like Luchang, Rachael struggled with depression and suicidal thinking and shared her fears on social media: "I have attempted suicide 3 times in the past 3 days and have not stopped thinking about it. What do I do? If I go to the hospital again this year, I will be academically withdrawn from my university. . . ." Days later, Rachael killed herself on campus.

This time, Yale students did not wait for the university to change its policies. A nonprofit organization named after Rachael (Elis for Rachael) and two current Yale students, Alicia Abramson and Hannah Neves, filed a federal lawsuit alleging disability discrimination. By publicly revealing their personal struggles and calling out Yale, Alicia and Hannah risked possible retaliation by the university, but their participation was critical. They established the required "standing" to sue, which would have been more difficult for an organization like Elis for Rachael.

Yale wisely chose to negotiate rather than litigate. A 2023 settlement agreement allows students seeking a voluntary medical leave the opportunity to discuss "potential accommodations that might allow them to remain enrolled." Yale can still order an involuntary medical leave, but only if the student poses a significant safety risk or is causing a severe disruption and "no reasonable accommodation can adequately reduce that risk or disruption." And in a reversal of policy, students on medical leave are now allowed to be on Yale's campus, though students living in on-campus housing must still move out. This is a significant change because excluding students from campus can cut them off from social support, thereby worsening existing mental health problems. The Yale settlement is an important victory, but the university should have made these changes much sooner. As noted earlier, the ADA has required reasonable accommodations since 1990, and fellow Ivy Princeton had settled a similar case with the Department of Justice in 2016. If Yale had acted earlier, it's possible Rachael's death could have been avoided.

The lessons learned at Yale go beyond medical leave to all aspects of education. Yale acted only after current and former students organized and filed a lawsuit. Two students publicly disclosed sensitive personal information to bolster the case. Change came from the bottom up, not the top down. The reforms sought were formulated by the students and their lawyers. Law professor Susan Stefan says, "the best solution is for the students themselves to get together to organize. . . . You understand it better than I do; you're there." She adds, "You're the ones who need to figure out what you need, and learn about the difficulties of negotiations with the powers that be."

In recent years, Yale has improved mental health services in other ways, including increasing capacity. But many Yale students say that they avoid seeking help because they fear being involuntarily withdrawn. This fear did not disappear the moment the case was settled. Perceptions can be more powerful than policy, and students understand that words on the page do not always translate into action. In contrast, students with mental health challenges can help one another without triggering negative institutional consequences.

Here's how Evan, who was considering withdrawal from college, explained it in a 2022 research article:

> *I needed a peer for school, I needed a peer. A friend who had been through the same thing I was about to go through perhaps because school's hard. This internship is hard and I was thinking, "Wow, if I don't make it past this first field work, I need to choose a new path maybe." My midterm was a failing midterm and ever since that, I got really anxious and really just, "I got to pass this." I was so scared that I would fail in this tiny frame of time. But it wasn't until my friend, who also failed—he's a year ahead of me. He reached out to me and he said, "And then I did it again and I passed with flying colors." Then I said, "Okay, so I should not be ashamed. I should not be scared. I can still do this. I don't have to go back home."*

Evan's experience is not unusual. The available evidence suggests that student peer support can be effective. A 2022 review article concluded: "Overall, studies suggest that peer support is associated with improvements in mental health including greater happiness, self-esteem and effective coping, and reductions in depression, loneliness and anxiety." Peer mentors can also benefit from the relationship. In one small study, mentors reported improvements in these areas, as well as increased feelings of empowerment.

Student peer mentoring programs come in many different shapes and sizes. One promising model is Project LETS. Peer mentors offer one-on-one support in "daily management, social/emotional support, linkage to clinical and community resources, crisis support, and ongoing support." Mentor training includes basic peer support principles, and also "trauma-informed care," "cultural dynamics," and "power and privilege." Since 2013, Project LETS has served over four thousand peers in over fifty high schools and colleges. The program is run entirely by individuals with lived experience. Applications by non-peer psychology majors who find mental illness "fascinating" are politely declined.

Stefanie Lyn Kaufman-Mthimkhulu founded Project LETS after her friend Britney died by suicide during Stefanie's freshman year in high school. The school district seemed more interested in sweeping the incident under a rug and avoiding liability rather than acknowledging that "something . . . really impactful had just happened." The silence lasted years. The deceased student's parents were unable to convince the high school yearbook to include their daughter, even when they offered to pay for a memorial page advertisement. The high school had guidance counselors and social workers, but there was an understanding among students that these professionals would report back to parents. It felt to Stefanie that students were on their own: "holding the space for each other with nothing but . . . our instincts and our love for each other." By the time Stefanie graduated from high school, she had a website and was running a live chat by herself.

Stefanie incorporated Project LETS as a nonprofit organization just before starting at Brown University. She also decided to go off all of her psych medications cold turkey. She struggled with withdrawal and told her professors. She was immediately called into student services, which knew about diagnoses she had not disclosed to her professors or to the school and asked if this was really a good time for her to start college. She felt trapped. Project LETS would train peers to become an independent resource for students who were looking for something other than just medication and therapy. Through Project LETS, peers learn about a college's resources, but the goal is not always a referral to traditional, non-peer providers. "I did not have a great relationship with Brown," Stefanie admits. She proposed a formal peer counseling program at Brown as a more sustainable option. After a year of Stefanie's time and effort, the director of the counseling center said no: "too risky, too much."

Stefanie decided to put together her own curriculum and run Project LETS independently. Administrators, therapists, and other students told her what she was doing was illegal—pretending to be a licensed therapist. One administrator told her that they would never put two depressed people together because they would just depress each other more. Undaunted, around sixty students signed up for the first training. But Brown would not provide physical space on campus for the trainings.

Around this time, a Brown student killed themself by jumping off the library. Brown reacted slowly, and poorly, according to Stefanie: "The only thing that they did was reroute the tours that were happening on campus so that all the new students and new families who were there just didn't see. They didn't walk past the library. That's how they responded." Project LETS filled the gap, posting on Facebook, communicating directly with traumatized students, and ordering pizza. A Brown administrator called Stefanie in tears, thanking the project for responding and asking how the school could help.

This was when the Brown chapter did its first suicide memorial. Stefanie explained, "Every year in the fall, we have folks kind of come and write messages to folks that they've lost to suicide and they speak and share stories and it's turned into this, like beautiful community space." The event celebrates survival as well by encouraging individuals to honestly share their struggles on a "failure confessional" board. Stefanie gave a couple examples: being rejected from every internship, or being in a psych ward all summer while friends traveled through Europe. Both the memorial and the board are powerful examples of peers shifting the narrative in positive ways.

Project LETS remains a grassroots organization. Its chapters have never been supported financially by the institutions. Volunteers continue the work on many campuses, but the organization has moved away from the chapter model. When we spoke in 2024, Stefanie told me about an educational program Project LETS ran in a Providence-area high school. The curriculum addressed stigma and marginalization, along with mental health awareness. Project LETS has also pivoted to focusing on crisis response. Stefanie gave one example of a student who was involuntarily hospitalized at Bellevue Hospital: "We have folks in New York who were there the next day doing an in-person visit and making sure they had their needs met." Project LETS is compiling an oral history archive of over one hundred people who have been involuntarily hospitalized. Like many, Stefanie uses the term "psychiatric survivors."

"Peer support" programs can look radically different than Project LETS. One of the oldest and most well-established peer support programs is the "Middle Earth" hotline at the University at Albany (State University of New York). Participation is not limited to individuals with lived experience, and the goal is to encourage students who may be struggling to connect with the professional counseling program. Longtime director Dolores Cimini emphasized that students are not "counselors" engaged in ongoing support but are instead "navigators." The program places navigators strategically to reach students who may be at higher need for help and lower likelihood of seeking it. The navigators are paid. The hotline advertises itself as "anonymous," but will employ phone-tracing in rare emergencies, with notice to callers that it is doing so.

Lean On Me is a national nonprofit organization that provides a school-specific encrypted text line for confidential nonclinical mental health peer support. Started in 2016 at the Massachusetts Institute of Technology, Lean On Me connects individuals experiencing distress with others in the same boat: "not someone throwing you a lifejacket, but someone who is in the same sinking ship," CEO Daniel Mirny explains. Sinking is hopefully an exaggeration, but the goal is "shelter in the storm," not easy solutions and sunny skies. Lean On Me provides peers with extensive training. Insurance is the program's biggest expense, though emergencies are rare. Crisis transfers make up less than half a percent of the texts. A dozen schools have now implemented the program. The fact that Lean On Me assumes legal liability has no doubt played a critical role in the program being adopted by so many colleges and universities. Recall Brown's reluctance to support Project LETS.

* * *

People with mental illness not only receive education, they provide it. No degree is required; experience is the best teacher. And the most traumatic experiences are often the most powerful. In general, people without a mental illness have not been confronted by a police officer during a crisis. They have not spent time in locked psychiatric facilities. They don't know how little mental health treatment is provided in jails and prisons. They haven't needed to navigate byzantine and overlapping disability benefits programs. They are less likely to be without health insurance or housing. There is no substitute for hearing directly from people with experiences like this who are now stable enough to tell their stories.

Remember Shannon Pagdon? She eventually broke free from her cycle of low-paying jobs, like barista and ice cream scooper, and finished her undergraduate degree at the John Jay College of Criminal Justice. When I spoke to Shannon in 2024, she was excited to be starting graduate school at the University of Pittsburgh—first to obtain a master's degree in social work, then a PhD. The holistic education program at Fountain House was critical to her success, but even more important was being part of a community of people with similar experiences.

Shannon shared with me something her experiences had taught her:

A lot of times, especially with supported education and employment programs, we kind of push people into getting jobs immediately, even if those jobs are very low-paying. I would argue that higher wage jobs are actually much less stressful. There's a lot less flexibility that one is given in low-paying jobs.

Even the best education programs may underestimate students' potential and be satisfied with them quickly clearing a low hurdle instead of stretching for a higher one. Many low-paying jobs are more stressful than high-paying jobs that require higher levels of education. Education can not only increase pay, but can also lead to more options, including a job that a person with a mental illness is more likely to keep.

This seemed like such an important insight that I did some follow-up research. It didn't take long for me to find this sentence in a 2024 article in *Psychological Medicine* (the second-most-cited journal in psychology):

Instead of rapidly placing service users from disadvantaged backgrounds in low wage, contingent jobs, we might instead engage more deeply with the structural origins of such factors as low self-esteem, lack of education, and uneven early work history, working to overcome rather than reinforce stratification, for example, by plotting a potentially slower path to further education and a living wage.

There's a reason why this sentence sounds so much like Shannon: She is one of the authors.

TAKEAWAYS

- There is no upper limit on educational and professional attainment for people with serious mental illness.
- The onset of mental health symptoms often interrupts high school and college.
- There are well-established but underused evidence-based programs to support students with mental illness.
- Some interventions save more money in government benefits than they cost to implement.
- Peers can provide essential support to other students.

PART III
Cure

CHAPTER 9

ADVOCACY

Jim Gottstein has devoted his career to improving mental healthcare in Alaska. He helped to create many peer-run organizations and innovative treatment facilities, including Alaska Mental Health Consumer Web, Mental Health Consumers of Alaska, Peer Properties, Inc., and Soteria-Alaska, Inc. (more on Soteria below). Jim has been building better community resources at the same time he was trying to tear down forced treatment by the state.

Inspired by Bob Whitaker's book, *Mad in America*, Jim founded the Law Project for Psychiatric Rights in 2002. The idea was to plan and then execute a "strategic litigation campaign" against abuse in the mental health system. An unexpected event forced Jim to cut short the planning phase and get straight to work. In February 2003, an acquaintance of Jim, Faith Myers, was involuntarily committed to the Alaska Psychiatric Institute (API). She refused medication. Jim began representing Faith in March 2003.

Faith had first been hospitalized with psychiatric symptoms in 1981, but she was doing well enough in 1999 to run a group care home for children. That changed when Faith started a new antipsychotic medication. She began hearing commanding voices for the first time in her life. A replacement medication worked better, but made her "terribly obese" and diabetic. Faith did not want to be medicated at API in 2003. The trial court acknowledged that Faith had articulated "a reasonable objection to the proposed medication," even as the court held that she did not have sufficient mental capacity to make her own treatment decisions.

A note on strategy: Jim may not have been able to control the timing of the cases or the characteristics of his clients (the cases were "somewhat random"), but he could select which arguments to raise on appeal. He generally limited himself to state constitutional arguments. The Alaska Constitution has relatively broad language protecting individual rights, language that sometimes mirrors statutory protections. Courts try to avoid constitutional rulings if the case can be decided on statutory grounds. Legislatures can change the outcome by passing a new statute. By pressing the constitutional claim, Jim did not give the Alaska Supreme Court and legislature that option. The state could not reverse a favorable rule based on the constitution with mere legislation. Using this strategy, Jim achieved longer-lasting victories.

One of those victories was in Faith's case on appeal. Based on the Alaska Constitution's express protections for "liberty" and "privacy," the Alaska Supreme Court in 2006 ruled for Faith in an opinion that set one of the highest standards in the country for forcible medication. The court declared that "the right to refuse psychotropic medication is a fundamental right," which can be overcome only by an independent judicial determination that medication is in the best interests of the patient and the least intrusive means. Faith was able to attend the oral argument and reports that Jim was "brilliant."

Jim is fueled by his own lived experience. He once jumped out of a second-story window to escape the devil. It was the middle of the night in 1982 but, as Jim tells it, he hadn't been sleeping at all for several days. The dislodged window hit the ground before he did. Unlike the window, Jim was fine. He ran across the street, frantically looking over his shoulder for the devil. What he encountered instead was a straitjacket, a ride to the state psychiatric hospital, and a forced injection of something that put him to sleep. When Jim woke up, they asked him what day it was. He couldn't answer, because he didn't know how long he had been asleep. To his captors, this was further evidence that Jim was disconnected from reality. That's also how many at the hospital interpreted Jim's seemingly grandiose, but true, claim to have graduated from Harvard Law School: just another delusion.

Hospital staff told Jim that he had a permanent condition and would never get better. The staff members who believed Jim when he said he was an attorney told him he'd never practice law again. After Jim was released, his psychiatrist had a much different view: Extreme sleep deprivation could drive anybody "crazy," so Jim just had to learn how to manage his sleep. He's even figured out the progression of symptoms that come before sleeplessness. The first one is not being able to finish sentences; next comes paranoid thinking. At that point, Jim will take a sedating medicine that provides "the most delicious sleep"; one night is usually enough to break the cycle. It's been five or six years since he's needed the medication.

Stress is another trigger. Lawyers cannot avoid hard deadlines, particularly in litigation. To reduce last-minute stress, Jim almost always files his pleadings, briefs, and other documents on the day before the deadline. The hardest part of this approach for Jim has been letting go of perfectionism. No brief is perfect, so you can always make it better by reviewing it again and again for another twenty-four hours, right up to the deadline. Filing early meant embracing the concept of "good enough"; "I'd like to think my good enough is pretty good." Jim has control over his time because he opened his own practice.

*　*　*

The depression following my first manic episode was almost unbearable. I had fallen so far and so fast with no guarantee I would ever get better. I was afraid I would kill myself. I didn't want to die, but after experiencing psychosis, I didn't trust my mind anymore. The delusion that I controlled everything (see chapter 1) was long gone. So, I controlled what I could. I stayed out of the kitchen because I thought I might cut myself with the knives. I avoided our twelfth-floor windows, fearing I might jump. And although I got better, that kind of fear doesn't ever go away completely; a part of me is still in that apartment. My advocacy comes out of that dark place.

A decade later, I was a law professor sitting in an auditorium listening to Supreme Court Justice Elena Kagan tell a story about going hunting with the late Justice Antonin Scalia. It was a funny story, but it reminded me that I needed to come up with a paper topic for a symposium on the Second Amendment. I had been invited to the symposium because of an article I had written with a former student, Amanda Adcock Young, provocatively titled "Do the Mentally Ill Have a Right to Bear Arms?" In other words, can the state prohibit gun possession by people with mental illnesses? Under the U.S. Supreme Court's case law at the time, the answer was not entirely clear (it still isn't). What *was* clear is that suicide prevention is the strongest argument in favor of restricting firearm possession by people with mental disorders. Most serious mental illnesses carry a substantially elevated risk of suicide. Violence toward others, especially mass shootings, may dominate the headlines, but the empirical link between violence and mental illness is relatively weak. People with mental illness are much more dangerous to themselves than to anyone else. And many of us know it, or at least I did after conducting research for the article.

As Justice Kagan spoke, I was thinking through the categories of people prohibited by federal law from possessing firearms. What was missing? That's when a simple idea struck me: People like me who fear suicide should be allowed to prohibit *themselves* from purchasing firearms. After my epiphany in the auditorium, I was only half-listening to Justice Kagan. I was giddy with excitement as I left the room. The idea felt like an unearned gift. Beyond keeping myself alive, I knew essentially nothing about suicide prevention. It felt like I had skipped the long process of becoming an expert and pulled a novel policy solution out of thin air. But in reality, I had much to learn before I could know if it was a policy solution that would actually be effective. At that moment, the only basis for the idea was my fear of what my own mind could do. So, I started at the end with the "Voluntary Do-Not-Sell Firearms List" (now generally known as Donna's Law) and worked backward through the research.

I had written many academic papers before—and I have written many more since—but writing that first article on this topic was a unique experience in my career. The path forward was wide open and straight. Every source I consulted provided additional support for the idea and its lifesaving potential. From at least the moment Ulysses tied himself to the mast to resist the Sirens' song, people have recognized the value of self-restriction. All the modern empirical research suggested that gun suicide would be an effective application of this principle. Suicide is very often impulsive, and the vast majority of survivors do not eventually die in a subsequent suicide attempt—90 percent choose to live. Firearms rarely offer a second chance, unlike other common methods. It was almost eerie how easy it was to write the paper.

That first article helped me get tenure. It's even been cited a few times in other law review articles. But for me, that paper was just the beginning. The empirical case was strong, but indirect and suggestive. It was a completely new idea and therefore completely untested. Feeling lucky to be a law professor who can do a little math, I set out to answer two key empirical questions: (1) Would anyone other than me sign up? and (2) Would signing up actually prevent suicide?

To get at these questions, the idea first had to be made more specific. A key dimension was (and remains) duration. Self-restriction could last for the rest of a participant's life, for a set period of time, or until some other condition is met. I decided that self-restriction should be reversible in order to increase the proposal's chances of being adopted, but to prevent impulsive gun purchase and suicide, there would need to be a delay period before reinstating a participant's ability to purchase a firearm. That, in effect, is an optional "waiting," or "cooling-off," period. At various points in time, many states have required that a purchaser return to the store some number of days after the purchase to take home a new gun. Other states require a permit or license to possess a firearm. Obtaining the permit or license takes time, so that also slows down gun acquisition.

So, one way of answering the second question—would signing up actually prevent suicide?—is to look at the success of waiting periods in reducing suicide. Do these mandatory across-the-board firearm purchase delays reduce suicide? Or do people just wait them out or switch to another method? At first, it was shocking to me to discover that I could find only one empirical study of the impact that waiting periods have on firearm deaths. It covered only explicit "waiting periods" during part of the 1990s. Three economists and I did a more rigorous study covering twenty-five years and all types of purchase delays. Consistent with all the other research about restricting access to suicide methods, purchase delays significantly reduced gun suicide without any increase in non-gun suicide.

Around the same time, I worked with a different team of researchers to anonymously survey two hundred individuals receiving psychiatric care. We asked participants if they would sign up for a program like this, if given the option. Some of my collaborators were skeptical. They figured very few people in progun Alabama would agree to restrict their own firearm access. Given my own experience, I was more hopeful. I guessed that maybe 15 percent to 20 percent of respondents would want to participate. We were all wonderfully wrong: 46 percent of respondents said they would sign up.

That's the moment I realized the idea really could save many lives. Delays work, and people want them. Existing law did not permit self-restriction, so we needed new legislation. You might think that a lawyer or law professor would know how to get a law passed. I didn't. So, I started trying everything I could think of. I pitched the idea directly to organizations (including the National Rifle Association [NRA]), experts, and policymakers. I wrote an op-ed that was published in the *Washington Post*. I was sure legislators would read the op-ed, be persuaded, and quickly enact the proposal. Needless to say, that didn't happen. Legislative advocacy is painfully slow.

***

Our indomitable Alaska attorney Jim Gottstein loves to "sue the bastards" (his words), but he recognizes that litigation alone has limits as a strategy to effect policy change. Faith's case was about involuntary medication, but the same general principle applies to involuntary hospitalization. The state can impose this extreme deprivation of liberty only if it is the "least restrictive alternative." Jim argued in a later case that his client could be successfully treated at Soteria-Alaska, a community residence with no physical restraints and little or no medication.

Soteria-Alaska (which Jim founded) had operated successfully for several years, but it was closed at the time Jim's client was committed. Soteria-Alaska may have been a "less restrictive alternative" when it was open, the court suggested, but Soteria was no longer "actually available" or "feasible"; "The State had no duty to re-open the private facility or to establish and operate a similar facility to meet its burden in this case." This reasoning may seem perfectly logical, even inevitable, but the ramifications are enormous. The state can effectively sidestep its legal obligation to place individuals in the least restrictive appropriate setting simply by choosing not to create or maintain any less restrictive settings. This problem exists across many areas, but the impact on people with mental illness is profound. The same dynamic pushes people into hospitals and assisted outpatient treatment when less restrictive community-based options could have been equally or more effective.

Another drawback of litigation as an advocacy tool is the personal cost. Plaintiffs in these cases are often vulnerable. The favorable ruling in Faith's case came at a very high price. When she began litigating, the retaliation was swift and severe.

> *They took away all my privileges, which really were rights. They took away the right to go to the gym, the right to go to the cafeteria. I had to eat my flavorless meals on the unit. They didn't even give me condiments. . . . I couldn't go outdoors in the middle of June and July. Everyone else was enjoying the outdoors, and I was stuck inside the unit.*

While the case was pending, API was prohibited by a court order from forcibly medicating Faith. However, if there is an "imminent threat of harm," then a facility is permitted to forcibly medicate a patient. "Every little incident" suddenly became an emergency. Here's how Faith describes what happened next:

> *Off to the room, lay me over the box, take down my underwear, and give me a shot in the bottom and to me that was like rape, because I had been raped two times in my life. And with these men surrounding*

me and holding me down and everything. It was like rape every time they did it. I was traumatized.

This trauma was compounded by systematic and appalling violations of privacy. Male staff members would enter unannounced into the women's bedroom, bathroom, and shower areas. Nowhere felt safe.

Winning her case did not improve Faith's life outside the facility, at least not immediately. She had alienated her family and had nowhere to live. It gets cold in Alaska. Her father died on her birthday, and she was unable to go to the funeral. She was too deep in mental illness. At least twice Faith was apprehended by police, one time resulting in a criminal charge. Eventually, she ended up back at API. This time she voluntarily took her medications—"Don't call Jim!" she told the staff—hoping finally to find a medication that would work for her. That happened right before she was released when they gave her a long-acting injection. The "delusions disappeared"; the "voices stopped." "And that's when I really started to be able to advocate, because I was in my right mind."

It may seem ironic that the woman who established the right to refuse psychotropic medication in Alaska only got better when she decided to take it. But Faith and Jim were not really fighting for or against medication; they were fighting for the right to choose, and not to be subjected to violence or retaliation for making the "wrong" choice. Standing in the light, Faith reached back into one of her darkest places: the trauma she experienced when male staff violated her privacy and her body. What the staff did was all legal at the time. Faith decided to change that.

Her goal in a new bill was to prevent others from experiencing the same kind of trauma. But, at a deeper level, it was about reclaiming autonomy and dignity for people in psychiatric facilities. First, the bill gave mental health patients at hospitals the right to choose the gender of any staff member providing "intimate" care. The hospital must inform patients about this right with a conspicuous notice. The second part of the bill required hospital staff to respect patient privacy more broadly, especially in same-sex bedrooms, bathrooms, and shower areas. Every psychiatric hospital and every state agency opposed it. All the advocacy groups lined up in support, providing letters and testimony. Stories like

Advocacy

Faith's carried the day, David beat Goliath, and the bill became law in 2008.

* * *

The people with the most power over public policy are our elected officials. Having elected officials who have had personal experience with mental illness might result in better mental health policies. But, historically, candidates for office have been punished for disclosing mental health problems. Perhaps the highest-profile example is U.S. Senator Thomas Eagleton. In 1972, Eagleton was forced to withdraw as a candidate for vice president after just eighteen days on the ticket when his history of hospitalizations for depression became public. It is impossible to know how many candidates after Eagleton kept their mental health diagnoses secret or decided not to run. Often forgotten, though, is the fact that Eagleton went on to be reelected to the U.S. Senate by Massachusetts voters twice after his disclosure.

There has been significant progress since Eagleton, and it appears to be accelerating. In 1994, candidate Lynn Rivers spoke publicly about her bipolar diagnosis while running to represent Michigan in the U.S. House of Representatives. Rivers not only won that election, but was reelected three times. Rivers was the first openly bipolar member of Congress. Congressman Seth Moulton began representing his Massachusetts district in 2015. He has spoken publicly about having PTSD as a result of his military service. It is not a coincidence that Moulton was a cosponsor of the bill establishing the 988 mental health hotline. In April 2019, Moulton announced that he was running for president. Like Eagleton, Moulton withdrew from the race for national office only a short time later (four months). Unlike Eagleton, Moulton's mental health diagnosis seems to have had little or nothing to do with his decision to withdraw from a crowded Democratic primary field.

In 2023, U.S. Senator John Fetterman of Pennsylvania publicly announced that he was admitting himself to the hospital for depression. The media coverage was intense. Fetterman did not resign. To the contrary, Fetterman's announcement garnered bipartisan praise, and he received an ovation from colleagues when he returned to the Senate floor. As we've seen, Fetterman is not the first politician to publicly and courageously discuss their own mental health problems. What's new, and hopeful, is the overwhelmingly positive reaction Fetterman received.

* * *

Disclosure is a risk for everyone with mental illness, not just politicians. My first psychiatrist in Alabama told me flatly not to disclose my diagnosis to anyone. "It could destroy your career," was his argument. I'm sure he gave the same advice to all his patients who were lucky enough to be able to conceal their diagnoses. It is true that the law provides special protections for job applicants and employees with known disabilities, but those protections are weak and under-enforced (see chapter 7). Discrimination is much more common. Hiding one's disability may achieve better employment outcomes than disclosure.

But hiding one's diagnosis has its own costs. It can cause stress and anxiety at work and lead an individual to avoid social contact with coworkers. Sometimes it's the concealment, not the symptoms of the mental illness, that lead to isolation, poor performance, and termination. Outside the workplace, an individual trying to keep their condition secret may choose not to apply for disability benefits or connect with formal and informal support systems. I once attended a National Alliance on Mental Illness (NAMI) peer support group while trying to hide my diagnosis. I quickly realized that meaningful participation would be impossible without disclosure. I didn't go back for years and lost that opportunity for peer support.

Instead, I followed my psychiatrist's advice not to tell anyone about my illness for many years. Carrying the weight of such a big secret was hard. My anxiety was exacerbated by the fact that my scholarship and teaching were centered on mental health law. It felt deceptive to present a case study as "hypothetical" when in fact it was based on one of my own experiences.* The irony, of course, is that my personal experiences

---

* In one article, the "hypothetical" case was exactly what happened to me: being "voluntarily" admitted to a psychiatric facility without the mental capacity to make that decision.

with the mental health system made me better at my job, not worse. I could see and feel things that outside observers could not. Still, fear for my career kept me in the closet. I could write "This happens, trust me," but I couldn't write "I know this happens because it happened to me."

In the end though, the personal costs ended up being higher than the professional ones. Students in my mental health seminar would disclose their own mental health struggles, or those of close family members. It was sometimes physically painful to suppress reactions like "I know how that feels" and "I've been there, it gets better." Still fearful after tenure, I finally disclosed my diagnosis to the dean and warned him that I planned to share my story with students. I felt a great weight lift.

The response from my seminar students was overwhelming and positive. More of them shared their own stories and our conversations deepened. It was a couple years after I started disclosing to my seminar students that I began disclosing my diagnosis on the first day of my two large lecture classes: Property and Trusts & Estates. Unlike in the seminar, my illness was not closely related to the subject matter. I did it because I wanted my students to know that a serious mental illness is nothing to be ashamed of and does not have to short-circuit a successful legal career.

I thought that disclosure would be like pulling off a Band-Aid: one and done. It wasn't. I have had to peel off the Band-Aid over and over, and it mostly sticks back on again. After you're functioning well, people don't seem to talk about your mental health nearly as much as you think they might. Of course, telling one student my diagnosis probably means that the whole law school quickly knows it. But the word "bipolar" covers such a broad range of experiences that no one knows my story until I tell it to them. The upside is that I get to pick and choose how, when, and what to disclose. For the first few years, I advocated for Donna's Law without telling my own story or revealing my own diagnosis, but I discovered that studies and statistics were not going to be powerful enough to advance the bills. It was time to rip off the Band-Aid in front of strangers.

November 16, 2017, was a cold day in Boston, but the hearing room in the capitol building was hot and crowded. The joint committee was considering a slew of gun-related bills that day. When at last it was my turn to testify, I started with the grim statistics on gun suicide and a description of the bill. I took a deep breath and continued:

> *What if the Commonwealth of Massachusetts passes the bill, but no one signs up? That's not going to happen. I know this for personal and empirical reasons.*
>
> *I have bipolar disorder. I've been suicidal. I want to sign up. Fifteen percent of people with bipolar disorder die by suicide. If I had had easy access to a gun at certain points in my life, I'd already be one of them.*
>
> *People who have never been severely depressed cannot understand what it's like. You lose joy, you lose hope, and you lose the ability to make rational decisions. However, like almost all people with mental illness, I have periods of clarity. During these periods, I want to protect myself against future dark days. . . .*
>
> *Help us help ourselves.*

For advocacy, disclosure can be a powerful weapon. Seconds later, I would learn that grief can be even stronger.

Andrea Scopelitis lost her son Joseph to gun suicide in 2016. With remarkable poise in that hearing room, she told his story. Still a young man, Joseph had battled severe mental illness for years. He bought a gun intending to kill himself, but his parents discovered the gun in time to prevent an attempt. They went back to the gun store, and every other gun dealer in the area, begging them not to sell him another gun. The same gun store that sold him the first gun sold him another. It would be his last purchase. Andrea and I had lunch together after the hearing. I learned more about Joseph, his struggles, and the almost superhuman ways in which his family had tried to take care of him over many years. They had done literally everything they could to treat his illness, to make him happy, and to keep him safe. More than a year after her son's death, Andrea's grief was still raw. It was the most powerful emotion I had ever seen another person experience, and it still is. I had been working for years on suicide prevention with no understanding of its full impact.

Advocacy

In spite of my efforts to personalize my arguments, and in spite of Andrea's moving testimony, the Massachusetts bill never made it out of committee. Just a few months later, though, a bill cleared all the hurdles in Washington state and was signed into law in March 2018. Three months later, in New Orleans, Donna Nathan bought her first firearm and used it to kill herself that same day. Donna and her family had been waging a heroic battle against her bipolar disorder and suicidal thoughts. Several times in the months leading up to her death, Donna gave up essentially all her rights by voluntarily admitting herself to psychiatric facilities, but there was no way for Donna to give up her right to buy a gun after being released.

Katrina Brees, Donna's daughter, was quick to recognize this gap and shared her frustration on social media. A New Orleans *Times-Picayune* journalist who had previously interviewed me about my work on the proposal in Alabama introduced us. Without the introduction, Katrina and I almost certainly wouldn't have crossed paths. She is an artist and Mardi Gras parade organizer; I am decidedly less interesting. Our differences haven't held back our partnership on Donna's Law, which continues to this day. The victims of suicide obviously cannot advocate for themselves. And the vast majority of people who have lost loved ones to suicide understandably do not want to share their story publicly. It is not fair to ask survivors to shoulder the burden of advocating for change. But Katrina didn't need an invitation. She has decided to tell her mom's story as many times as it takes to give others the lifesaving option of suspending one's own ability to buy a gun.

Katrina and I ramped up our efforts to enact bills in all fifty states, with help from too many people and organizations to count.[*] I have

---

[*] I do not mean "countless" figuratively; no list of key contributors could be exhaustive at this point. With apologies to many, I will list just a few: John Autry, Ian Ayres, Bryan Barks, Rosemary Bayer, Rob Bonta, Ken Buck, Heidi Campbell, Jennifer Chan, John Curtis, Marjorie Decker, Vicki Doudera, Steve Eliason, Heather Elliott, Phillip Ensler, Allen Farley, Diane Feinstein, Nicole Gibson, Chloe Grabowski, Will Guzzardi, Jimmy Harris, Lee Harris, Pricey Harrison, Morissa Henn, Shelly Hettleman, Gigi Thompson Jarvis, Pramila Jayapal, Nathan Johnson, Robyn Kennedy, Cathy Kipp, Raja Krishnamoorthi, Taylor Kleffel, Mandie Landry, Mary Lee, Patty Lewis, Virginia Mack, Doug Mann, Sarah Marshall, David Meuse, David Moon, Eric Morrison, Jarrod Ousley,

elsewhere described some of the ups and downs we encountered in various states. In 2020, after years of falling short in other states, Virginia became the second state to enact the proposal. I testified in Richmond right before the pandemic. Both Katrina and I testified by Zoom in Utah, which enacted its version in 2021. Delaware was the next state to enact Donna's Law, in 2024, and Colorado in 2025.

***

"Nothing about us without us."

Judi Chamberlin popularized this rallying cry among mental health advocates. Her 1978 book, *On Our Own: Patient-Controlled Alternatives to the Mental Health System*, is a founding document of what would become the modern peer movement. Chamberlin's preferred term was "the mental patients' liberation movement," which was also the phrase used by an organization she cofounded in the early 1970s. In the book, Chamberlin describes her own traumatic involuntary hospitalizations in the 1960s and contends that the threat of force poisons the entire mental health system. Chamberlin's core argument is that patients must reclaim their autonomy. While the focus of *On Our Own* is on alternative treatments, peers who read it were empowered to demand broader policy reforms.

Chamberlin was not the last peer author-turned-advocate. Diana Chao attempted suicide shortly after finding out that she had bipolar disorder. She was only thirteen years old. Her parents had immigrated from China and spoke no English. The family lived below the poverty line. Without access to traditional mental healthcare, Diana coped by writing letters to no one in particular. She found her own voice and realized that she had a story worth telling. In 2013, Diana started a small club at her high school centered on that idea. "Letters to Strangers" (L2S) has

---

Elena Parent, Darisha Parker, Stephanie Pasternak, Brooke Pinto, Trip Pittman, Jamie Pedersen, Neil Rafferty, Dan Rayfield, Liddy Renner, Tina Riley-Humphrey, Beth Joslin Roth, Lindsay Sabadosa, Kim Schofield, Reed Shafer-Ray, Ed Stafman, Jennifer Stuber, Scott Surovell, Vernon Sykes, Yusi Wang, the American Foundation for Suicide Prevention, and the National Alliance on Mental Illness.

become the "the largest global youth-run nonprofit seeking to destigmatize mental illness and increase access to affordable, quality treatment, particularly for youth," with over one hundred chapters in seventy-two countries. The organization has expanded well beyond letter writing—it now gives scholarships and advocates for legislation. This rapid growth was fueled primarily by the internet; the book came later. In 2019, L2S published the *Youth-for-Youth Mental Health Guidebook*.

Social media also makes it possible for an individual to be an advocate without any organizational support. The irrepressible Samantha Smith (see chapter 7) is one such advocate. In a popular social media post, Samantha offered advice about how to maintain mental health during election night. Samantha now posts about mental health on Instagram about once a day. She also sends emails to state legislators and has met with some of them in person.

Nor was Judi Chamberlin the first person diagnosed with a mental illness to write a book about their experiences in psychiatric facilities or to found an important advocacy organization. Not even close. Seventy years before Chamberlin's book, Clifford Beers's 1908 autobiography, *A Mind that Found Itself*, had outlined abusive treatment inside public and private psychiatric hospitals. The next year, Beers cofounded an advocacy organization that is now known as Mental Health America (MHA). MHA remains one of the most important organizations dedicated to mental health policy. Among many other accomplishments, MHA played a key role in passage of the Protection and Advocacy for Individuals with Mental Illness (PAIMI) Act. The PAIMI Act is all about ensuring representation of peers in oversight and decision-making.

To influence policy and its implementation, there is no substitute for having a seat at the table where the decisions are made. That often happens below the level of elected officials. In 1986, responding to Connecticut Senator Lowell Weicker's investigation into hospitals abusing and neglecting people with mental illness under their care, Congress passed the PAIMI Act. The Act expanded the scope of existing state-level protection and advocacy programs, which had previously been limited to serving people with developmental disabilities. An important feature of the PAIMI Act was the creation of an advisory council in each state overseeing professional advocates. At least half of the council members were required to be "individuals who have received or are receiving mental health services or who are family members of such individuals." That percentage was later increased to 60 percent and had to include the council chair.

The PAIMI program has achieved some important successes. A 2011 independent evaluation concluded that "PAIMI programs provide those with psychiatric disabilities a voice in the exercise of their rights, and they are highly successful in achieving client and system goals and objectives." Their policy successes included: (1) being "instrumental" in enacting psychiatric advance directive laws in a number of states; (2) playing a sometimes "very significant" role in legislative examination of mental health parity; and (3) getting legislation to divert individuals out of jail and into treatment. To be clear, state PAIMI programs vary widely in effectiveness, and nearly everyone agrees that these programs receive insufficient funding.

Another way peers can change policy is by working within government agencies. In the late 1980s, Alabama led the way with the nation's first senior administrative position expressly reserved for a peer and dedicated to bringing that perspective to the table. Joel Slack was the originator of the idea and the first director of the office within the state mental health agency. This model was widely copied. By 2010, over forty states had an Office of Consumer Affairs (OCA).* Some of these offices were involved in senior management and policymaking, whereas others focused on consumer complaints. The overall trend is encouraging, but six offices were vacant, three were housed in a contracted organization, and at least ten had no budget-making authority. Of course, having no permanent home within the agency and having no say in resource allocation decisions limit substantially the potential of OCAs to impact policy.

Not even embedded and empowered OCAs are secure. Recall the landmark *Wyatt* litigation in Alabama that recognized for the first time a federal constitutional right to adequate treatment for involuntary

---

* Recall that "consumer" was once the preferred name for people receiving mental health services. Some still prefer that label.

hospitalized psychiatric patients (chapter 2). Through a combination of improvements and a massive number of patient discharges, the state, after thirty-three years of foot-dragging, finally complied with its treatment obligations in 2004. U.S. District Judge Myron Thompson therefore dismissed the case, declaring:

> *Today, as a result, any judge, legislator, or executive official who would seek to reverse the everyday involvement and oversight of state and local advocacy groups, friends and family members of people with mental disabilities, and self-advocacy by consumers of mental-health care, would face universal condemnation. This legacy of this litigation cannot be terminated by any court.*

Half of this prediction turned out to be true. In the twenty years since this order was entered, no court has overturned the key holding from the *Wyatt* case that states have a constitutional duty to provide adequate treatment to psychiatric patients held against their will in state facilities. Peer involvement and oversight has actually been less secure in recent years, at least at the federal level.

Donald Trump does not bother to conceal his disdain for people with disabilities. Indeed, as a presidential candidate in 2015, Trump once publicly mocked a physically disabled *New York Times* reporter, even mimicking some of the movements caused by his condition. Many people expressed outrage, but Trump nonetheless went on to win the 2016 election. His assault on people with disabilities carried over into policy. This included eliminating the federal office responsible for peer involvement and oversight. Trump kicked the peer perspective out of the room, reversing this legacy of the *Wyatt* case.

When Paolo del Vecchio joined the Substance Abuse and Mental Health Services Administration (SAMHSA) in the mid-1990s, he was the first person there to self-identify as a person with a mental health history. Paolo has openly discussed being restrained by police officers during a mental health crisis and the resulting "shame, fear, and pain." When interviewed about the new 988 mental health crisis number, Paolo emphasized that the overarching goal is a "full continuum of recovery-based and trauma-informed care." People often end up in crisis due to problems with "social supports, housing, or job stress." Before and after the Trump administration, Paolo has helped shape countless policies affecting people with mental illness. Trump pushed Paolo into the background.*

Early in his presidency, Joseph Biden brought Paolo back and put him in charge of a newly established "Office of Recovery." The peer voice was represented again, for the time being. One of the top priorities of mental health advocates during the Biden administration was to make sure future presidents would not be able to turn back the clock so easily. Congress considered a bill to protect the gains made by peers. The PEER Support Act would codify the Office of Recovery and require that its director have "demonstrated experience in, and lived experience with, mental health or substance use disorder recovery." It may seem strange to enact a bill "establishing" an office that already exists, with a well-qualified director like Paulo. But if the PEER Support Act had been passed, a future president would not have been lawfully able to eliminate peer representation at such a high policymaking level without another act of Congress.

In the first few months of the second Trump administration, half of the Office of Recovery staff were laid off. Paolo left (or was forced out) in March 2025. Paolo did not go quietly into the night. In April 2025, he wrote:

> *At the age of twenty-three, after years of mental health problems, addictions, and trauma, I found myself on a Philadelphia subway platform ready to end my life.*
>
> *Thankfully, I found help and got better. But due to the actions of the Trump administration, many others face a bleak future in dealing with these potentially fatal conditions. . . . In just three months, Trump and Kennedy have dismantled 30 years of federal mental health and substance use leadership. . . .*

---

* A leading advocate in Alabama, Jon Brock, pointed to Trump's actions as strong evidence of Paolo's bona fides and effectiveness.

Advocacy

> *We need SAMHSA and the important programs it supports so that others can find recovery like I have and live healthy, happy, and productive lives in our communities.*

A leaked budget draft put a target around the entirety of SAMHSA's budget. But in May 2025, Trump proposed cuts of over $1 billion to SAMHSA's $8 billion budget. Back from the brink of total elimination, the fate of the Office of Recovery is still unclear.

In contrast, in a first-of-its-kind bill passed in 2024, Washington state solidified its commitment to peer participation in policymaking. The rationale stated in the bill is as simple as it is radical: "People with direct lived experience with a particular issue are experts in their own lives and experience and are best equipped to find solutions to those issues." The law requires that all multimember legislative task forces and advisory committees include at least three individuals with lived experience. Not some task forces, all; not one member, three.

The origin story of the Washington bill demonstrates the power of the lived experiences it protects. A group of self-advocates conceived the bill and led the charge. Ivanova Smith, who has mild intellectual and developmental disabilities, was a leader of the group. Smith has explained that the law will not kick any experts out of the room; instead, "we're saying let's extend the table, let's put in more chairs. . . . I need to hear from the experts, but the experts need to hear from me." This commitment to inclusion runs deep in the disability rights movement.

The name of Washington's new law is the Nothing About Us Without Us Act.

* * * **

A federal bill could enact Donna's Law in every state all at once. That's why I spent years searching for a sponsor in Congress. Our successes at the state level turned out to be essential to finding sponsors in Congress. Seattle-area Congresswoman Pramila Jayapal learned about the proposal because it had passed in Washington. In 2018, Jayapal's office reached out to Jamie Pedersen, who introduced me in turn. And it was not by chance that one of the two Republican cosponsors in Congress was from Utah, another enacting state. For well over a year, I worked closely with Jayapal's office to refine the language of the bill. Then, it was a matter of waiting for a window to introduce the bill when it would have a chance of success.

Representative Jayapal introduced the bipartisan bill in Summer 2022, but she did not push for a hearing until the lame-duck period after the November election. This seemed like good timing because Democrats still controlled the House, and the NRA said that it would remain neutral on the bill. Even though Republicans were in the minority, their opposition could run out the clock on the session. Two days before the hearing, the NRA reversed its position and announced its opposition. The Republicans on the committee dutifully lined up in a row against the bill. The federal bill passed out of committee on a party-line vote, but there was no chance of moving it quickly enough to pass over Republican opposition. This was one of our hardest losses. We knew the chance of passage in Congress was small, but the payoff could not have been higher.

This was neither the first time that the NRA thwarted our efforts, nor would it be the last. It seems that the NRA wants to promote gun sales and does not care how the guns will be used. In opposing Donna's Law, the NRA has abandoned its professed commitment to individual liberty in favor of paternalism with respect to people who might voluntarily choose self-restriction. The choice not to buy a gun deserves as much protection as the choice to buy a gun, unless of course the goal is to sell guns and not to respect individual choices. Ideological incoherence is frustrating, but the NRA's attitude toward people with mental illness is even more offensive.

A representative of the NRA asked one of our state sponsors: "How can a person with a mental condition give away their rights?" But having a mental health diagnosis does not mean a person lacks mental capacity. Every day, people with psychiatric diagnoses get married, make binding contracts, execute their wills, and waive constitutional rights.* There's another problem with this line of argument. Suppose an individual, with

---

* We also write books like this one.

or without mental health issues, does not have the mental capacity to sign up for Donna's Law. Would we trust that same person to buy a gun? Again, it's symmetric—a person either has the mental capacity to make a decision about gun possession or they don't. What isn't symmetric is the cost of getting this decision wrong: Mistakenly allowing a person to sign up for a gun purchase prohibition creates, at most, a twenty-one-day delay to buy a gun; mistakenly preventing a person from signing up can be fatal.

Sadly, the NRA doesn't need coherent arguments to control Congress and many state legislatures. The NRA masterfully employs a wide variety of tactics. Obviously, it makes substantial campaign contributions to candidates who commit to oppose any gun regulations. On the flip side, the NRA withholds, or threatens to withhold, contributions from legislators who support gun regulations. The organization sometimes shifts its support to a more "progun" challenger in the Republican primary. And their support carries great weight with voters and the party. Without spending any money, the NRA can lower a politician's letter grade on its well-publicized list—being downgraded from, say, A to B could tip the next election.

The NRA doesn't always wait for the next regularly scheduled election. When I initially contacted a public health expert in Colorado, the first thing he said was that there would be no chance of passing any gun-related legislation for a long time. He explained that in 2013 the NRA had orchestrated successful recall campaigns against two Democratic state senators who voted for gun regulations after a series of mass shootings, including one in Aurora, Colorado. No one in the legislature was going to touch guns. And though it did take a very long time, Colorado eventually passed Donna's Law in 2025.

**

There are many different ways to be an advocate. Misperception and fear drive policy. After a mass shooting, the NRA almost invariably blames mental illness to distract attention from the firearm or firearms used. This, along with other factors such as media depictions, has contributed to the pervasive myth that all people with mental illness are dangerous to others. Challenging negative perceptions of people with mental illness is critical both in passing reforms and in preserving them. Against the backdrop of discrimination and shame, disclosure alone can be a powerful tool.

There is room for quiet advocacy as well. One of the most powerful and private places a person with mental illness can make a difference is the voting booth, but equal access to the voting booth cannot be taken for granted. Many states prohibit individuals from voting solely because they are under guardianship, without any individualized consideration of a person's mental capacity to vote. One advocate estimated in 2018 that at least 32,000 people in California were disenfranchised on account of guardianship laws during the preceding decade. Other states have only recently abandoned even less defensible restrictions. For example, before a 2010 amendment, the New Mexico Constitution prohibited "idiots" and "insane persons" from voting. Offensive and vague restrictions like these still appear in the laws of many other states.

The Arizona Constitution provides that "no person who is adjudicated an incapacitated person shall be qualified to vote at any election." At a guardianship hearing, Annette Wood, who had been diagnosed with dementia, admitted that she needed help making medical decisions, but argued that she was still able to vote. The judge found that Wood hadn't met her burden to prove that she had "sufficient understanding to exercise the right to vote." The appellate court reversed and held, as a matter of federal constitutional law, that the party seeking guardianship must bear the burden of showing Wood lacked sufficient understanding to vote. A guardianship order, standing alone, does not eliminate the presumption that an adult has the mental capacity to vote. Everyone starts with the right to vote.

And with the right to vote comes untapped power. Two Rutgers University professors, Lisa Schur and Douglas Kruse, estimated that if people with disabilities, including people with serious mental illness, voted in 2020 at the same rate as people without disabilities, there would have been about 1.75 million more voters. But increasing turnout affects the outcome only if people with disabilities vote for one candidate more than for the other. During the 2020 campaign, candidate Trump made no secret of his personal antipathy toward people with disabilities, even publicly mocking a disabled reporter. And in contrast to Biden, Trump promised to repeal the Affordable Care Act (often called "Obamacare"), which greatly expanded mental health coverage and protections. Economic and cultural issues appeared to have driven votes for Trump, but it is still somewhat surprising that people with disabilities split evenly.

The National Disability Rights Network offered this explanation:

While 81 percent of voters with disabilities considered it very important for candidates at both the congressional and presidential level to address issues important to people with disabilities, only 41 percent could recall hearing, seeing, or reading about anything from the candidates about disability issues. In battleground states, where political advertising and voter outreach is more common, that number drops to 33 percent. Given that 50 percent of voters with disabilities said that the candidates' stances on disability issues strongly impacts their vote, the apparent relative lack of outreach signals a missed opportunity.

It was not just the candidates who missed an opportunity; voters with disabilities may have missed the opportunity to educate themselves about the two candidates. Another explanation for the even split is that people with disabilities, like most people, are not actually single-issue voters. People with mental illness have multiple identities, just like everyone else (see chapter 11). Still, learning more about candidates' positions on issues affecting people with mental illness and factoring those positions into voting choices could determine outcomes in close elections.

* * *

People with mental illness have been advocating for change for a very long time and in many different ways that have changed the world for the better for those of us with mental illness. We are survivors, litigants, lawyers, lobbyists, organizers, educators, role models, witnesses, elected and appointed officials, insiders, outsiders, and authors. Few of us will be heroes like Judi Chamberlin, Jim Gottstein, or Faith Myers. But luckily there are many other ways for regular people with mental illness to be advocates. Simply telling even one other person about your diagnosis can help fight negative stereotypes. Learning about the issues and voting can make a huge difference. It will take the combined effort of all of us to keep moving forward.

TAKEAWAYS

- People with mental illness shape policy in many ways.
- Filing lawsuits and enacting new legislation can change one law.
- Running for office and voting have the potential to change many laws.
- Being in the right room and speaking out can be powerful.
- Reducing stigma is required for systemic and lasting change.

CHAPTER 10

HUMANITY

A person with a mental illness is a person. This proposition is true as a matter of logic, but it's difficult to reconcile with the United States's response to mental illness. The response in this country is almost purely medical. A person is reduced to their diagnosis, and the only prescription is medical treatment, by force if necessary. And even medical treatment is largely reserved for those lucky enough to have health insurance that will pay for it. We provide inadequate healthcare and fail to provide for other basic needs. Even if medical care were a panacea, accessing consistent medical care is nearly impossible without food, housing, a job to pay for housing, and transportation to the clinic. These basic needs are rarely included in the U.S. approach to mental illness. But if a person is fortunate to have these essentials, survival may be the best a person with mental illness and limited privilege can expect.

Creating a meaningful life is about more than meeting basic needs. A person with a mental illness, like every other person, deserves an opportunity to create the life they want: to become part of a community, to go to school, to get a good job, and to feel good about themselves. If this list sounds familiar, that's because it is the same for people without mental illness. Everyone has multiple identities and the potential for growth. Recognition of shared humanity is the crucial first step toward sustained improvement in the lives of people with mental illness.

* * *

Black people have been fighting for equality in the United States since they first arrived in 1619. It was a fight they did not choose. Slavers in Africa had violently robbed them of all liberty, put them in chains, packed them into ships, took them across the ocean, and forced the survivors to work. The Black experience in America is both unique and universal. This country's history of racial oppression and courageous resistance is unlike anything else. But one critical step in any fight for human rights is convincing the people in power that members of the disfavored group are, in fact, people. Only humans have human rights.

An assertion of shared humanity has always been central in the fight for racial justice. In 1857, the U.S. Supreme Court in *Dred Scott v. Sandford* held that a slave taken into a free state was not a "citizen" and therefore could not file a lawsuit in federal court. In the majority opinion, Justice Taney referred to enslaved people as "a subordinate and inferior class of beings." Two justices dissented: "A slave is not a mere chattel. He bears the impress of his Maker, and is amenable to the laws of God and man; and he is destined to an endless existence."

It took the Civil War and a constitutional amendment to vindicate the dissent in the *Dred Scott* case. That victory would prove to be short-lived. Adopted in 1868, the Fourteenth Amendment says that states cannot deny any person the "equal protection of the law." Rather than follow this clear mandate, the Supreme Court in *Plessy v. Ferguson* (1896) adopted the "separate but equal" doctrine to uphold racial segregation. In his dissenting opinion, Justice Harlan wrote: "The law regards man as man." After almost sixty years of state-sanctioned segregation, the Supreme Court finally held in *Brown v. Board of Education* (1954) that separate is "inherently unequal."

But judges cannot remake society. Black people continued to demand justice, and the Civil Rights Movement gained momentum. In his famous "Mountaintop" speech on the night before he was assassinated, Martin Luther King Jr. described some of the movement's goals: "We are saying that we are determined to be men. We are determined to be people. We are saying that we are God's children. And that we don't have to live like we are forced to live." In 1968, King was demanding that Black people be recognized as human, in almost exactly the same words as the dissenting justices in *Dred Scott*, well over a century earlier. As demonstrated by the Black Lives Matter movement and the tragic events that sparked it, that's still a core demand.

King was in Memphis that night to support a sanitation workers' strike. Economic justice was a new front in the Civil Rights Movement. Every person deserves a good job. But the first battle is still to be counted as a person. What did all the protest signs say during the Memphis strike?

"I AM A MAN."

At least five years earlier, patients at mental hospitals had made the connection between the Civil Rights Movement and their own struggles. In June 1963, Vivian Malone Jones and James Hood, backed by threat of force from a federalized national guard, walked through the doors of Foster Auditorium and became the first Black students to register at the University of Alabama. Governor George Wallace's infamous stand at the schoolhouse door had failed.

At that moment, less than a mile away, around five thousand people were locked behind another door. As discussed in chapter 2, Bryce Hospital was one of the oldest and largest state-run inpatient psychiatric facilities in the country. One journalist described it as a "hellhole." Photos showed patients strapped to rocking chairs. There were only three psychiatrists: one for every 1,700 patients. State expenditures per patient were at or near the lowest in the country.

Here, we see two types of buildings: buildings people want to get into and buildings people want to get out of. In both cases, equality can be achieved only by opening the door. The struggles and successes of patients at Bryce are far less well known than the events across town, but they are connected in deeply important ways.

One perhaps surprising connection happened almost immediately. The evening after the drama at the schoolhouse door, President John Kennedy delivered his famous address on civil rights. The next morning, June 12, 1963, Medgar Evers, a Black leader involved in desegregating the University of Mississippi, was assassinated. On July 6, 1963, the patient-edited newsletter at Bryce reported that "about 175 persons did what was called a memorial march Sunday for the slain Negro [Medgar Evers]. It was all quiet and peaceful."

As of 2023, Bryce Hospital had just 268 beds. Thousands of people have made it out of that locked door. Deinstitutionalization has obviously been controversial. Support for individuals in the community has been inadequate. But allowing individuals with mental illness to live free of unnecessary restraints is a profound recognition of liberty, equality, and shared humanity.

I <u>AM</u> A PERSON.

I do not mean to overstate the analogy between mental illness and race. Most people with a mental illness would rather not have it. Symptoms can be painful, disabling, and even deadly. Life would be harder for a person with a mental illness even in a world without stigma and discrimination. In contrast, racial hierarchies are based on arbitrary differences. "White" is better than "Black" only because racist White people had the power to impose that view. Still, there are deep connections between the struggle for Black civil rights and for the rights of people with mental illness. At bottom, both are premised fundamentally on the view that all people deserve equal concern and respect, including basic human rights.

* * *

On the first day of every class, I tell the students that my experience with bipolar disorder inspired a suicide prevention proposal. In Fall 2024, I was able to follow up with: "The Governor of Delaware signed my bill this morning!" The students all clapped, which felt great, but my goal in beginning every semester this way is to challenge negative stereotypes and to connect with students who may be struggling. Difference is worth celebrating if it is employed to good ends.

Since I started disclosing my diagnosis, many students have opened up to me about their own struggles. One wanted advice about how to answer the discriminatory and illegal mental health questions on the Alabama bar application. Another wanted to tell me about the suicidal crisis that landed her in the emergency room the week earlier. My hope is that many more have felt validated and encouraged just from knowing I am a professor at their law school. At a minimum, all my students see an older authority figure demonstrate that a mental health diagnosis is not something to be ashamed of or hidden. I go into greater depth about my personal experiences in my mental health law seminar. Because of the nature of the class and the focus on mental health, my seminar students also hear me tell stories of vulnerability and resilience, both my own and those of people I interviewed for this book.

To be sure, disclosure is a two-edged sword. I am frequently invited to speak about mental health and firearm law, and I often testify when my proposal is introduced in a state legislative committee. In a recent session with medical students, I asked them what they thought about my decision to disclose my own diagnosis (chapter 9). One student expressed the view that the rest of my testimony might be discounted as that of a "crazy person." Perhaps, I thought, but then I considered the context. My testimony begins with my fancy academic title, and it includes hard statistics. At hearings, there are almost always other people testifying as well with complementary messages, but rarely someone who can explain why they want to sign themselves up. Demonstrating that there is real demand for the proposal is important because enrollment has been relatively low in the enacting states. But these maybe are rationalizations. Either way, I felt the student's comment like a gut-punch. It was painful to be dismissed out of hand like that and even worse to recognize that it happens to people with serious mental illness all the time.

* * *

"Stigma" is the word most commonly used to describe negative perceptions about people with mental illness. One problem with the word "stigma" is the way it deflects responsibility from the bad actor. "Racism" is the word for the abhorrent views held by "racists." Racism, the idea, is not the problem; the problem is that so many racists believe it, and act on it. There is no word like "racist" to describe someone who believes in or acts on "stigma." "Stigmatizer" is never going to take off, even if it is an actual word. Without a good noun for the actor, the passive voice is unavoidable. The guilty party is invisible.

Another problem is vagueness. When the word "stigma" is used in the context of mental illness, it sometimes describes negative perceptions, but other times the term also includes negative actions based on those perceptions. Here's one example: Stigma is defined as "the prejudice and discrimination attached to devalued conditions." Despite these shortcomings, it is too late to replace "stigma" with another word. It has become the standard term, both inside and outside academia. Plus, there is no obvious alternative. I believe the umbrella term "stigma" consists of five separate ideas that are often (but not always) lumped together: difference, disdain, discrimination, dehumanization, and demonization. The focus of this chapter is on the beliefs and actions of non-peers. The related phenomenon of self-stigma is examined in chapter 11 ("Identity").

Difference. Whether or not negative perceptions lead to discriminatory actions, the prerequisite for all stigma is a perception of the difference itself. This perception can arise from merely knowing or suspecting an individual's diagnosis or from direct observation. Mental illness often has a recognizable impact on behavior. That almost inevitably leads to categorization. By virtue of visible symptoms, one group appears to have a mental illness, one group doesn't. That's just a difference, which in theory could be neutral. People with mental illness are not mind readers, so mere negative perceptions do not have any direct impact on them. Different negative perceptions lead to different types of discrimination, but actions are what matter at the end of the day.

Disdain. Mental illness is generally considered abnormal and undesirable, so the perception of difference can quickly turn into disdain. Mental illness is bad, society believes, so people who have a mental illness are not just different, they are worse. Familiarity with mental illness may reduce disdain. Friends and family see the whole person, not just a diagnosis. But many people don't have the opportunity to have a close relationship with a person with serious mental illness. Portrayals in the media are overwhelmingly unflattering. Highly successful people with mental illness tend not to disclose their diagnosis, whereas dramatic failures make headlines.

One way disdain manifests itself is in a desire for social distance. In a 2018 survey of the U.S. general population, over 60 percent of respondents expressed unwillingness to "work closely with" a person with schizophrenia. That number had not changed significantly since 2006. More hopeful, the comparable percentage for depression fell from around 45 percent in 2006 to around 25 percent in 2018. But a quarter of the population is still a huge number of people. Lower, but still substantial, percentages of respondents were unwilling to have as a neighbor, socialize with, or make friends with people with either schizophrenia or depression.

Discrimination. These negative attitudes translate into significant hurdles for people with mental illness. Disdain fuels housing and employment discrimination. Landlords are less likely to indicate property availability if an applicant discloses that they are "receiving mental health treatment in a hospital." One British survey of eight hundred persons in mental health advocacy groups found that "more than a third had been terminated from jobs." These examples of discrimination are common, but there are also examples of discrimination that are far more severe and disturbing. The prevalence and severity of observed discrimination against people with mental illness suggests that "disdain" is only the beginning, and there are other forces at work.

Dehumanization may be a more accurate term. "Disdain" implies that people with mental illness are "less than" people without a mental illness, at least in some important respects. But "disdain" implies that they are still people. In contrast, dehumanization is the belief that mental illness deprives a person of their humanity. One who suffers from mental illness is "less than" human in every way. In this view, having a mental illness means having no rights that people with mental illness are obliged to respect. Mass hospitalization, incarceration, and homelessness are evidence of dehumanization; mere disdain would not seem powerful enough to account for the general public's acceptance of the status quo in these areas.

Demonization justifies the worst type of discrimination: overusing force. This can take the form of police abuse, arrest, or worse. Recall from chapter 1 Laquan McDonald, who was shot by police sixteen times while walking away from them. But force can manifest at various points in an individual's lived experience: ejection from homeless shelters, inappropriate involuntary hospitalization, forcible medication, and so on. To be sure, not every use of force is illegitimate, but force should always be the last resort. Demonization predictably leads to force more often than it is required.

* * *

Demonization and the fear that comes with it is the most powerful component of stigma and the justification for the most severe mistreatment. Over 60 percent of the general population believes that people with schizophrenia are dangerous toward others, a number that has barely budged in the last two decades—in fact, it is creeping up slightly. Fear of individuals with depression is shared by a remarkable one in four Americans. At some level of perceived risk, the public will demand force and coercion as a means of collective self-defense.

To be clear, a person with schizophrenia, especially during a first psychotic break, is more likely than other people to commit an act of interpersonal violence. But the absolute risk of harm is vanishingly small—on the order of a lightning strike. Most people with serious mental illness have prolonged periods without symptoms, or with only mild symptoms, during which they are no more dangerous than anyone else. Even people during crises pose a very low absolute risk of violence. Recall from chapter 1 how few police officers are killed responding to mental health calls, as compared to how many mentally ill individuals are killed by police. One summary of eleven studies estimates that society would have to detain thirty-five thousand high-risk people with schizophrenia to prevent one homicide against a stranger. Fear is an irrational response to this level of danger, yet it is still pervasive.

The media and entertainment industries play a major role in creating and perpetuating fear of people with mental illness. One study of the period 1995 to 2014 found that 55 percent of four hundred randomly selected newspaper and major network TV news stories about mental illness mentioned violence, while only 7 percent told a story of successful treatment or recovery. The stories of violence and people with mental illness in newspapers have become harder to miss: Just 1 percent of these stories during the first decade of the study were on the front page; that figure was 18 percent during the second decade. Television and film are just as stigmatizing. A study of movies and TV shows in 2016 and 2017 found that 46 percent of characters with mental illness were perpetrators of violence.

Demonization can lead directly to force and coercion, the worst forms of discrimination—including violent police response to a crisis, unnecessary arrest and criminalization, physical restraint, and forcible treatment. Combating the perception of dangerousness should therefore be the highest priority of destigmatization efforts. Those efforts are not working. Among the general population of the United States from 1996 to 2018, "perceptions regarding potential violence and support for coercion generally rose over time—significantly so for schizophrenia. By 2018, over 60 percent of respondents saw people who met criteria for schizophrenia as dangerous to others, and 44–59 percent supported coercive treatment." The authors of the study conclude that large-scale anti-stigma efforts have been "a categorical failure."

Anti-stigma campaigns take different forms. Many campaigns prioritize education about the causes of mental illness, emphasizing the biological basis for the disease. The rationale is that this information would reduce negative judgments and increase empathy. But these programs appear to have reinforced difference and have not materially affected perceived dangerousness. Perhaps it should not be surprising that relabeling "mental illness" as a "brain disease" does not reduce stigma. The cause of the difference does not appear to affect society's negative perceptions.

Another anti-stigma strategy is disclosure by famous and successful people. An ever-growing list of celebrities and athletes are openly discussing their own mental health. For example, in May 2024, the entertainment website IMDb posted a list of 197 actors and celebrities with mental illness. The list is as diverse as it is long. A sample follows:

Alvin Ailey (dancer, choreographer, and dance company founder)
Buzz Aldrin (second person to walk on the moon)
David Beckham (legendary English soccer player)
DMX (actor and rapper)
Simone Biles (best gymnast of all time)
Stephen Colbert (comedian and talk-show host)
Sheryl Crow (Grammy-winning singer-songwriter)
Robert Downey Jr. (Oscar-nominated actor who plays Ironman)
Bill Gates (billionaire philanthropist and founder of Microsoft)
Michael Jordan (best basketball player ever)
Selena Gomez (singer and actress)
Jimi Hendrix (singer, songwriter, and guitarist)
Prince Harry (Duke of Sussex)
J. K. Rowling (billionaire author of the Harry Potter books)
Nina Simone (singer, songwriter, and civil rights activist)
Ted Turner (billionaire media mogul)
Mike Wallace (*60 Minutes* journalist)
Catherine Zeta-Jones (Oscar-winning actress)

Disclosure by a famous person obviously reaches many people at once, and a celebrity's well-known accomplishments can, in theory, call into question pervasive negative stereotypes about people with mental illness. In practice, however, celebrity disclosures do not appear to be working to reduce societal stigma.

But bigger is not always better. Small-scale disclosure may actually be more effective. Research shows that knowing a friend or family member with a mental illness reduces stigma. So telling even just one friend about your mental health struggles pushes public opinion in the right direction. Sure, celebrities can reach people more efficiently, but the number of these celebrities is microscopic in comparison to the millions of people with mental illness who are not famous. Indeed, research shows that celebrity disclosures are less impactful than disclosures by individuals who are more relatable to members of the audience. The combined impact of enough small-scale disclosures can surpass the effect of high-profile ones. To reduce stigma and to move public opinion forward, it will take disclosures both big and small.

It is not an accident that most celebrities wait until after they have achieved success to go public with their diagnoses. Celebrities have to make the same trade-offs as everyone else. The benefits of disclosure must be weighed against the costs. Discrimination and stigma are pervasive. That's why I waited until I had tenure before telling colleagues and students about my bipolar diagnosis. Before I testified in that crowded Massachusetts hearing room (chapter 9), I consulted with two successful law professors who were public about their diagnoses. Professor Elyn Saks of the University of Southern California was particularly encouraging, and inspiring. A fellow graduate of Yale Law School, Elyn is a leading mental health law scholar and a MacArthur Fellow. Elyn's life with schizophrenia was the subject of both her bestselling memoir, *The Center Cannot Hold*, and her wildly popular TedTalk, which has been viewed more than five million times since 2012. It's hard to imagine anyone more successful or more public than that (certainly among law professors!). I was extremely lucky: Very few people with serious mental illness have the job security and role models that I did. No one with a mental illness has any obligation to disclose. It's a personal and strategic choice that is not for everyone.

***

Direct contact with a person who has a mental illness reduces stigma. Structured and targeted disclosure on a small-scale has a stronger evidence base. Two programs in particular stand out. In Our Own Voice (IOOV) is an anti-stigma program developed by peers at the National Alliance on Mental Illness (NAMI). In thirty- or ninety-minute sessions, two trained facilitators with lived experience discuss five stages of their recovery: (1) dark days; (2) acceptance; (3) treatment; (4) coping mechanisms; and (5) successes, hopes, and dreams. Research finds that IOOV improves the ratio of positive to negative perceptions of people with mental illness. Other studies confirm reduced stigma. In addition to combating public stigma, the program aims to give hope to peers and their families.

Facilitators report that the IOOV experience was "healing and empowering." One peer put it this way in an IOOV video: "Getting these emotions out with another person who you know has worn your shoes, has walked your path, just gives you that energy, gives you that hope."

Mental health providers often hold the same dehumanizing stereotypes as the general public. These unconscious and conscious negative perceptions held by providers can result in substandard treatment, misdiagnosis, and other negative outcomes. NAMI has developed an anti-stigma program aimed directly at providers. The NAMI Provider program is intended to foster a greater understanding of the lived experiences of the family and individual in order to encourage more empathetic and collaborative care.

The five-session program is co-led by a person with direct lived experience, a family member, and a provider. Marilyn Roberts, a family-member instructor, she explains the importance of contact: "That lived experience piece is like . . . gold. It is the one thing that changes people's opinions and removes that bias. . . . Every single one of them that stands up and talks . . . is chipping away at that bias that people with lived experience are not productive, [that] they can't work, and that they're a burden on the system." Providers tend to see patients in crisis much more often than patients who are doing well. Interacting with a person with serious mental illness that is living well in recovery allows providers to see beyond the crises, to the whole person.

NAMI Provider uses an evidence-based curriculum designed to put providers into the shoes of their patients. The "hearing voices exercise" sometimes moves provider-participants to tears. These participants are asked to complete a simple task while simultaneously listening to intrusive audio of voices talking in their ear. The voices can be merely distracting observations about the weather or threatening statements like "these people are out to get you."

Family-member instructor Leslie Carpenter recalled a provider-participant approaching her after the hearing voices exercise and saying, "I had never stopped to think about how difficult it is to even have a conversation while you've got thirty voices in your head talking at you at the same time." Leslie went on, saying "they had just never thought of it, right? And why would they? It's not part of the typical didactic training. Sure, they know that people have auditory hallucinations, but they never stop to consider what the experience is like for the person."

Another Provider program exercise is focused on the stigma attached to different diagnostic labels. Provider-participants hold a sign with a specific diagnosis like schizophrenia, bipolar, or depression. The other participants are instructed to write down their first unfiltered thoughts about people who have that diagnosis on Post-it notes and to stick the notes to the back of the providers holding the signs. The gut reactions are very often negative—like "crazy," "unstable," and "lazy." Each participant is asked how it feels to hear negative perceptions about their condition and how it might feel to be treated this way. The second part of the exercise then requires them to place positive and empowering words on each person.

NAMI Provider has been shown to successfully improve the beliefs, attitudes, and perceptions held by heath care professionals, which consequently improves care for those individuals living with severe mental illness. Studies have highlighted that, when implemented into a medical school curriculum, the program has a significant positive longitudinal impact. Specifically, up to six months post-intervention, student-participants reported less stereotyping, stigma, and anxiety surrounding patient interaction, as well as increased confidence, competence, and collaborative care skills.

* * *

Stigma begins with a perception of difference. Peers look for and see similarity, not difference. In this most important way, peers cannot help but recognize each other's humanity. We are not "other" to each other. Of course, no one's story is the same, but all of us have experienced some symptoms of mental illness. Peers do not disdain, dehumanize, or demonize one another. As a result, peers can push back against stigma more effectively than others, whether or not they disclose their own diagnosis. All people with mental health challenges deserve support, not disdain. People with mental illness have the same basic needs as everyone else, especially during more difficult phases of the illness.

Quality healthcare is a basic need, but meeting even more basic needs can suffice to avoid tragic outcomes. Food is sometimes enough to avoid a potentially dangerous police encounter. Recall from chapter 1 Vania's experience responding to an individual in mental health crisis waving a knife. Her team de-escalated the situation in part by providing the man with snacks. Police carry guns, not snacks. Recognizing that a person in crisis still has basic human needs and prioritizing those needs comes naturally to peers.

Demonization is an especially pernicious type of stigma, and it is not limited to acute crisis response. Criminal legal involvement and mental health struggles can even be job qualifications. For example, personal experience is essential for peers in mental health courts. Justin Volpe had just graduated from the Miami mental health court in 2007 and was walking out of the courtroom for what he thought was the last time. He was excited to go celebrate his twenty-fourth birthday. That's when he was stopped and offered a peer position with the program. He said, "Lady, I'm paranoid. I'm delusional." Her response, "You'll fit right in." Justin took the job and went on to work in that program for fourteen years, helping over a thousand people. Justin is now senior peer support coordinator at the National Association of State Mental Health Program Directors (NASMHPD).

The stigma surrounding mental illness is unlikely to disappear any time soon. Large-scale anti-stigma efforts have achieved relatively small gains. Efforts to combat discrete discriminatory actions and policies may deserve greater immediate attention than attempts to change hearts and minds. That said, smaller-scale, targeted anti-stigma programs like NAMI Provider that rely on direct interaction with peers have shown promise. Involving peers at every stage of the illness and recovery process has the potential both to mitigate the impact of stigma right now, because peer providers are less likely to perceive clients negatively, and to break down stigma in the future, as success stories multiply.

TAKEAWAYS

- A sense of shared humanity is the key to overcome stigma and perhaps all social justice movements.
- "Stigma" is a combination of difference, disdain, dehumanization, demonization, and discrimination.
- Peers see sameness, not difference, and play a key role in anti-stigma efforts, big and small.

CHAPTER 11

IDENTITY

Hector Ramirez has had terrible experiences in hospitals. Once, he was furious when he woke up in a hospital three months after a suicide attempt. It was the fact of waking up that made him angry, not being in the hospital. Another hospital stay was far more traumatic. During a mental health crisis, a police officer took Hector to a hospital. He was handcuffed to a pole in what felt like a detention room. Still, Hector had one good thing to say about hospitals. It wasn't about the medical treatment, it was "being with the other patients, because it was nonjudgmental." He told me it was the only time he didn't have to worry about stigma, shame, and feeling like a burden to his family.

Being diagnosed with a mental illness can shatter any person's sense of self. Hector explains: "I don't hear anybody calling themselves mentally ill for fun. . . . It's not a positive thing." Putting the pieces back together is an important step in recovery. Without incorporating the diagnosis into a new, positive identity, that empty space fills up with shame, loneliness, and hopelessness. To be clear, the label causes its own harm in addition to the harm caused by the illness. That's because a person who receives a diagnosis has already experienced symptoms of the illness, and a mental health diagnosis is determined solely by a person's symptoms. Negative internal and external reactions to the new label often make the situation worse, at least at first, by lowering self-worth and healthy risk-taking, and by increasing paternalism and discrimination.

A negative sense of self caused by a mental health diagnosis is usually referred to as self-stigma or internalized stigma. There are many negative effects. Studies show that high self-stigma causes social withdrawal, decreases quality of life, and increases suicide risk. Clinical outcomes suffer, including more hospitalizations and suicides. Self-stigma can set off a vicious cycle by reducing functioning, which leads to poor outcomes in other areas of life, which in turn reinforce self-stigma. With such deeply ingrained causes and such a wide range of effects, no single intervention can be expected to solve the problem. You may be surprised by some of the things that have been shown to help: listening to music, playing soccer, flying in an airplane, and moving to Canada. We'll get to those later in the chapter, but first, more on the problem of self-stigma.

* * *

Upon diagnosis, the individual automatically becomes a "mental patient." Society views this identity negatively. To be clear, there is at least one practical advantage of getting a mental health diagnosis: opening the door to targeted medical treatments. As prior chapters discussed in detail, other consequences are less obviously positive. There are specialized courts, mental health courts to prevent individuals with mental illness from falling into the black hole of the criminal legal system. The insanity defense is supposed to do the same thing, but mostly doesn't (chapter 3). Similarly controversial, a person with mental illness can be hospitalized involuntarily, medicated forcibly, and compelled to participate in outpatient treatment (chapters 2 and 4). To receive other government benefits, a person must self-identify as "mentally disabled." That phrase triggers the protections of the ADA, including anti-discrimination and reasonable accommodations provisions (see chapter 7).

The words "patient," "ill," and "disabled" have strong negative connotations. An illness must be treated and fixed, generally by doctors. Having a disability means that the individual is less capable than other people in some significant way. Either framing can exacerbate self-stigma. In place of a medical framing (patient, illness) or a legal framing (disabled), some people prefer the terms "consumer" or "service user." These terms are neutral and intentionally vague (like "peer"). Eliminating any direct reference to mental illness or disability arguably reinforces the idea that the condition is shameful and should be kept hidden. Moreover, a person using these terms is defining themselves based on their relationship to the mental health system. For this reason, some advocates for systematic change use phrases like "psychiatric survivor" and "mad." The system or the society is the problem, not the individual.

Labels have personal as well as political significance. In an important sense, identity consists of the words a person chooses to describe themselves. Labels like "mental patient" and "mentally disabled" imply that the person has a problem for doctors to solve or is permanently defective. The result may be low self-esteem and resignation—sometimes referred to as a "victim mentality." A victim is not responsible for their condition and may therefore feel less responsible for their recovery. Giving up control can lead to giving up altogether. In contrast, "survivors" have endured hardship and shown strength. The "madman" doesn't care what you think about him; he's not bothered or held back by a society that wants to put him down.

In addition to labels, there are many other times when words convey messages that reveal the stigma of mental illness. "Put Alabama to Work" may seem like an appropriate name for an employment initiative for people with disabilities. But to peer specialist Christina Fox, it "sounded kinda negative." She explains: "Put them to work" implies that people dealing with mental illness don't want to work. That's a common misconception. "Help them to find work" is what Christina does every day. Clients set their own employment goals, and she helps them along. She provides support, not instruction. Recall Mike Autrey's definition of recovery from the introduction: "creating a life that you want." Not a life someone chooses for you. Autonomy is essential to recovery.

The words used to describe symptoms are also contested. Are Shannon Pagdon's voices "auditory hallucinations" or "lived experience of a nonconsensus reality" (her words)? Does the latter phrase demonstrate a "lack of insight"? Clinical labels cannot capture the nuances of individual experience, and many labels imply judgment. Sometimes, negative messages are expressed openly. To convey the seriousness of a new diagnosis and the importance of treatment, many healthcare providers tell patients explicitly to lower their expectations. Shannon asks, "If we are told by experts our lives will be hollow shells of our previous hopes and dreams, how do you start believing something different?"

Not all medical labels are bad, and some of the worst ones are being replaced. For example, a patient who fails to take their medication is now described as "nonadherent" rather than "noncompliant." Nonadherence is less negative than noncompliance. Compliance suggests that the patient must follow the doctor's orders, whereas adherence implies a somewhat greater degree of patient autonomy. Medical terminology can be useful for more than making treatment decisions. Some people endorse clinical labels and integrate them into a new sense of self.

Often, healthcare professionals make it harder for a patient to view themselves as more than a diagnosis. Understandably focused on symptoms and side effects, doctors can lose sight of the patient as a person—"There's a schizophrenic in room 5," for example. A patient who hears this kind of language may start to believe that they are nothing more than a diagnosis. And the doctors, as well as the rest of the healthcare team, can also lose sight of the humanity of the person in room 5. The problem is not limited to healthcare. Society sends powerful negative messages about mental illness. A person is defined by their diagnosis, and the diagnosis is shameful, debilitating, and dangerous.

There is an underappreciated relationship between psychiatric medications and identity. "Anosognosia" is another term for lack of insight. These terms are used to describe a patient who refuses treatment because the patient does not believe they have a mental illness. Refusing treatment by itself creates a presumption of anosognosia, and that presumption can be hard to overcome. If a person gives other reasons, the doctor may discount or ignore those reasons, or even consider them to be further evidence of anosognosia. For example, if a patient isn't convinced by the overwhelming evidence that the medication is beneficial for people with the same diagnosis, the only rational explanation is that the patient doesn't believe the diagnosis. To be clear, a lack of insight caused by mental illness can sometimes be the only reason for refusing treatment, but not always. There are many other logical reasons patients refuse treatment. Most psychiatric medications have only limited effectiveness, and even the most effective medications, like lithium, don't work at all for many patients. Other patients may decide that the side effects outweigh the benefits. Yet, when there is the possibility that a person may have anosognosia, it is easy for healthcare professionals to discount a person's autonomy and to view them as troublesome patients, not autonomous people.

Psychiatric medications may also create issues for people struggling with the "mental patient" label. Taking daily medication is a reminder that they are a "mental patient," by definition. Additionally, because psychiatric medications act on the brain, they pose a genuine threat to one's sense of self. Is this the real me or is this the drugs? Some people who accept their diagnosis stop taking medications just to be able to answer this question. Even medications that have significant clinical benefits can exacerbate an identity crisis in a person who is struggling to find or maintain identity in the face of mental health symptoms.

* * *

A new mental health diagnosis sets a person apart from everyone in their lives. The shock to identity is profound. The diagnosis doesn't change the person, but it changes the person's sense of self. It is almost like becoming a new person. Relationships must be redefined or rebuilt, and some people will cut all ties. Fear of social rejection can lead to isolation even without actual rejection. Sometimes, the separation is physical. A diagnosis may open the door to a hospital, then lock the door behind you. One way or another, the result can be profound loneliness.

Being alone forever is my greatest fear. I realized the depth of that fear on a locked psych ward. Perhaps because I had so much of it, I was obsessed with time. By far the most important time each day was when my wife Caroline arrived in the afternoon to visit. One morning, I saw the second hand stop on the wall clock in the cafeteria. I screamed. When a staff member rushed to replace the battery, the clock fell to the floor. In my mind, that meant Caroline would never come back, and I would be stuck alone in that space forever. I'd have rather died.

The best cure for loneliness is being with other people, but that's not the only thing that helps. Music helps me. Ten months after that clock stopped, Brandi Carlile released a song called "What Can I Say." It begins:

> Look to the clock on the wall
> Hands hardly moving at all
> I can't stand the state that I'm in
> Sometimes it feels like the walls closing in
> Oh Lord, what can I say?
> I am so sad since you went away
> Time, time ticking on me
> Alone is the last place I wanted to be

The song is about missing a loved one, but it means more than that to me. The lyrics describe the darkest moment of my life with startling specificity. But rather than making me sad or scared when I hear it, I feel less alone every time.

More and more songs have begun exploring mental illness directly. Selena Gomez spelled out in lyrics exactly what she hoped to accomplish with her 2022 song, "My Mind & Me":

> My mind and me, we don't get along sometimes
> And it gets hard to breathe, but I wouldn't change my life
> And all of the crashin' and burnin' and breakin', I know now
> If somebody sees me like this, then they won't feel alone now

Other artists go so far as to name specific medications that are effective for them—for example, Sting (lithium) and Kanye West (Lexapro).

Singer-songwriter Morgan Wade does not endorse any specific drug; instead, she encourages people to keep trying to find the right medication:

> By summer's end, I predict that I'll
> Have finally lost my mind.
> The doctor said that these new pills,

Well, they might help me this time.
And I hope that's the case 'cause I feel I am wastin'
The one life that I have.
The chances they come, and the chances they go,
But the time, well, you can't get that back.

This message is important because finding the right drug and dosage on the first attempt is extremely rare. Even more important is the broader message to start the recovery process sooner, not later. Many people with mental illness fear the future, but the passage of time is not always bad. Take, for example, these lyrics from Matchbox Twenty's 2003 song "Unwell": "I'm not crazy, I'm just a little unwell. I know, right now you can't tell. But stay a while and maybe then you'll see a different side of me." Mental health crises are temporary, and recovery is always possible.

Research confirms the power of music. One survey in the United Kingdom found that 80 percent of young people (fourteen to twenty-five years old) believe music and other live events improve their mental health. In April 2017, the hip-hop artist Logic released a song called "1-800-273-8255," which was the suicide hotline number at the time (it is now 988). A 2021 study examined the song's impact on calls to the hotline and the number of suicides. The researchers found significantly more calls and significantly fewer suicides in the days after the song's release and after two awards shows featuring the song. They estimate the song saved 245 lives. Music can be the difference between life and death. It can build a bridge between a person who feels entirely alone and ready to die and one empathetic listener who gives them back hope.

* * *

Every person has multiple identities, but some people have more identities than others. The difficulty of a puzzle goes up with the number of pieces. So, too, with identity. There are more categories to redefine, reprioritize, and rebuild, and they all have to be reconciled with each other. On the other hand, having many identities increases the chance that one of them is so sturdy that a diagnosis can't shake it. These identities won't have to be rebuilt and can provide a foundation for other identities. Intersectionality is a blessing and a curse.

Religion was clearly a blessing for Samantha Smith. Therapy had brought Samantha to accept and understand her depression, but it was religion that gave her hope and made lasting recovery possible. She reframed her illness as "an attack . . . from the enemy" and enlisted a powerful ally in the fight. "God wants me to be happy." Samantha is winning her battle. She has stopped taking antidepressants. She's not against medication in an emergency, but she wants to address her underlying issues without them. A healthcare provider might call this "nonadherence," but it is working just fine for Samantha.

Not every church supports people with mental illness. Christi Collins found that out the hard way: "Even though I was going to a church, that church pretty much threw me away after the suicide attempt. Well, you just should go to hell. You know, after such a thing." She eventually moved to a new church, where Christi runs a peer support group. The church had a tradition of bringing bring food to members on all sorts of occasions: a new baby, a battle with cancer, or a death in the family. Christi added mental health struggles to the list and gave the program the best name ever: "Where's My Casserole?"

Race complicates the experience of having a mental illness. Mental health stigma is stronger in the Black community. One study found that people who identified as Asian or Latino were significantly more likely than other races to think they didn't need treatment. White and Black respondents were more likely to cite stigma and wanting to handle it themselves. Preventing people who need help from seeking it is probably the most tragic consequence of stigma and self-stigma. Black people with less education reported more structural barriers than other racial and ethnic groups.

Within the system, however, sharing a racial identity can help create trust and connection. After Leslie Napper's first mental health crisis and still "not really understanding the system," she was assigned a White case manager. The case manager cried when Leslie told her about her struggles. Leslie assumed that her experiences must be "really bad," because they made even a professional cry. She stopped sharing her story with the case manager to avoid further harming either of them. When Leslie eventually switched to a Black case manager, they quickly established a trusting and supportive relationship. She was able to open up again. Leslie attributes her problems with the first case manager to implicit bias and a lack of understanding on both sides. They could not get over the racial divide: "I am Black and you are not."

Gender is another core identity that intersects with mental illness. Women with schizophrenia have different experiences than men with the same diagnosis. A 2023 article* reviewed the literature: "Studies show that women with schizophrenia experience greater illness-related shame than men, leading them to frequently hide their diagnosis, and that authorities often question their reports of victimization. In addition, women living with schizophrenia report experiencing paternalism and sexism." Providers sometimes tell women who have schizophrenia not to have children.

Ethan Frost has overcome steep obstacles to forge a positive identity. He was molested throughout his childhood, but the perpetrator was never prosecuted. Instead, the church pastor ordered therapy and counseling for the perpetrator. It turned out Ethan would be the one to go to jail. His conviction was for an assault he didn't commit, but he was at the scene and in possession of illegal drugs. He got time served and ten years of probation. Ethan's drug problems only got worse. At age thirty, he connected the dots between his childhood trauma and his struggles with addiction. Around that time, Ethan was diagnosed with substance use disorder, autism, bipolar disorder, and ADHD. Having multiple diagnoses is common. Each diagnosis introduces its own new component of identity, and many diagnoses have fuzzy boundaries and overlapping symptoms.

Somehow, Ethan put all these pieces together to form a new identity as a forensic peer specialist, helping people with the transition out of jail and prison. Drawing on his own experiences, Ethan solves practical problems for his clients, like getting identification, public benefits,

---

* If you have read chapter 7, you won't be surprised to learn that one of the authors is Shannon Pagdon, who is a woman living with schizophrenia.

housing, transportation, and employment. He describes some difficulties facing a person just released from jail or prison. You can't get housing without an ID; if you get an apartment, you won't be able to pay rent unless you have a job; without transportation, you can't get to a job, to a doctor, or to the probation officer; if you miss any those appointments, you are more likely to end up in crisis, hospital, jail, or homeless.

Along with Ethan's many other diagnoses, he received the one with the greatest impact on his identity: gender dysphoria. Ethan always knew he had been born in the wrong body, but he delayed transitioning because of the intense stigma in his community. "It's okay to be gay. It's okay to be lesbian. . . . But once you want to change your body into another gender, that's a whole different issue." Many people believe that challenging the male–female binary is both sinful and an attack on their own identities. Ethan had internalized the stigma and shame. When he eventually got up the courage to ask his doctor for hormone replacement therapy, the doctor not only refused, but fired him as a patient.

Ethan didn't give up. He found another doctor farther away. After starting hormone therapy, Ethan's mood was "100 percent better." He believes that transitioning has helped with "creating this identity of being sober too." Being trans is a foundation that Ethan is building on. I asked him how anti-trans sentiment compares to the stigma of mental illness and addiction. Both types of prejudice assume that there's a choice and that the root problem is a lack of willpower, he explained. "People believe that mental health is just your inability to manage your own life." The same false assumption applies to people who are transgender or suffer from substance use disorder.

The biggest difference, Ethan said, is that people who are anti-trans don't hide it. Negative comments about mental illness and addiction are often whispered behind closed doors, whereas anti-trans people are "very unapologetic and they're very in your face." When hate is so directly and forcefully asserted, it's easy for a person to start hating themselves. And when loved ones turn away, a person loses core identities like "child," "sibling," and "friend." When Ethan's family abandoned him, he didn't give up on himself. He's building a new family instead. As the interview was ending, Ethan told me he was about to get married. "Spouse" is one of the best identities.

Hector Ramirez is another remarkable example of intersectionality. Hector wanted to kill himself for years after the suicide attempt described at the beginning of this chapter. He was born in Mexico and identifies as "half native" (indigenous). Hector has been diagnosed with everything from autism to schizophrenia and bipolar disorder. He is also a gay man. Perhaps because of that identity, one psychiatrist in a public hospital refused to prescribe Paxil, which is the antidepressant medication Hector knew he needed and asked for by name. Instead, the doctor prescribed seven days of prayer. "Completely devastated," Hector went straight home and tried to hang himself in the backyard. Religion is a lifesaver for many people with mental illness, but one doctor twisted his own religious views into a weapon that nearly ended Hector's life. On another occasion, Hector had a seizure in that same backyard. A neighbor saw it happen and called 911. The responding police officer decided that Hector was dangerous, so the officer repeatedly slammed Hector to the ground, breaking his jaw and cochlear bones in his left ear. His hearing loss was permanent, so Hector learned sign language.

Hector later used this new skill, and remarkable courage, while pulling a hearing-impaired person out of a dangerous situation. During the rescue, the police hit Hector again, this time a literal shot in the back. It was the summer of 2020, after the Minneapolis police killed George Floyd, an unarmed Black man with mental health problems. Like many cities, Los Angeles erupted with racial justice protests, which started out peacefully but became violent in places. Upon learning that the mayor might shut down public transportation in response, Hector had to find another way. He had to help two disabled individuals get to the temporary shelter he had found for them. One of them needed sign language interpretation. As the protest spiraled out of control, he struggled to keep hold of "his guys." Then Hector was hit in the back by a beanbag that the police had fired into the crowd. But he stood up and kept struggling down the street. The bruise would be huge, but the pain that day did not stop Hector. They made it to the shelter.

IDENTITY

"I don't sit anywhere," Hector observes, referring to his overlapping and marginalized identities. But Hector can sit almost everywhere precisely because he doesn't sit anywhere. His résumé is eight pages long, including participation and leadership in five national, ten state, ten county, and seven city entities and organizations. Most of this work is centered on mental health, but other positions relate to health equity, education, and disability more broadly. Hector's multiple identities and singular history of trauma give him insights no one else has. He's in a dozen rooms using his voice to shape policy.

* * *

Peers supporting one another reduces self-stigma. Peer support can take the form of a one-on-one mentoring relationship, or a formal self-help group, or something in between. Over half a million Americans participate in self-help groups each year. With a formal group, every success by one member proves to the others that success is possible. Individual wins become wins for the whole group. Losses are easier to bear. There is encouragement after a setback by people who may have gone through the same thing. Members may even take more risks because they know they have a safety net.

Fountain House started in the 1940s as a self-help club and still embodies those principles. A self-help group provides a safe space for members to share common experiences and to provide and receive support from one another. Participation is voluntary, and the members control the group. There are many types of self-help groups. Mental health groups are common. Studies show that self-help groups improve participants' self-esteem, hopefulness, and sense of well-being. Members of peer groups feel validated and empowered. Longtime disability rights advocate Ann Marshall told me this about support groups: "I'm not sure there's an alternative or better way to kind of break down self-stigma."

The principle of peer control has spread well beyond self-help groups. Peers now operate their own drop-in centers, outreach programs, housing and employment assistance programs, crisis response teams, suicide hotlines, and businesses. Peer providers form positive identities around their new positions. Each position has a new label, like "peer support specialist," "program director," and even "CEO." "Mental patient" is not on the list.

Sometimes, an ongoing relationship isn't required to achieve lasting changes. Simply sharing space creates opportunities for people with mental illness to learn from one another in profound and unexpected ways. Cyrus Napolitano told me about one time he was leaving Fountain House:

> *I went to the receptionist desk [to swipe out] and there was an older Black woman there. I had seen her around the house. I think her name was Joan.* Now, Joan talked to herself. She was having conversations with people that weren't there. I remember she said, "Have a good night and God bless you." I said, "You too. Have a good night and God bless you too." And I started walking away, and she was having this conversation with somebody that wasn't there. And I stopped. And I started listening. Now I couldn't make out what she was saying, but that wasn't the important point. I was recognizing her as somebody with value, despite the fact that she was talking to somebody that I couldn't see. And it didn't bother me. I was like, "Oh, this is what it's like to have schizophrenia. . . . And I just stood there for a few minutes and it was like, it was just such a powerful moment because it's like wow, she's a real person, just like me. She has her challenges. She has her issues. She has her problems. You know what? So do I. It doesn't make me any better than her, and it doesn't make me any worse than her.*

Listening to another person with lived experience helped Cyrus recognize their humanity and intrinsic value, and his own.

Soccer is more than just a game. A 2019 Spanish study found that participation in an indoor soccer league for people with serious mental illness was associated with a significant reduction in self-stigma. Each of the fifteen teams played two competitive games a week for nine months

---

* Not her real name.

of the year. The players also helped run the league. The researchers concluded that "belonging to a specific and structured program with goals closely tied to the inclusive process and the participation of people with [serious mental illnesses] in the community through sports has a positive effect on decreasing internalized prejudice."

Some things are even more important than soccer. Ann Marshall is a pioneer of peer empowerment and disability rights. She told me two stories. The first was about a teenage girl who had been dropped off at Bryce Hospital as a very small child. After getting special permission to leave the hospital, the girl traveled in a van to a national disability rights conference in South Carolina. She was both "excited and terrified." The other twelve peers in the van took turns sitting next to the girl and holding her hand to keep her calm. She made it there and back, triumphant. The second story was also about travel. A man with a serious mental illness attended a different conference. He had never flown, never even left Tuscaloosa, but he bravely went all by himself. Ann recalled, "He was great, and he got on that plane, and it started flying away, and I started crying. I couldn't help it. I was just so impressed by his courage. You know, I think that's what kept you going, those kinds of things."

Taking risks and overcoming fears can be transformational. Applying for a job can be intimidating for anyone, but the potential payoff is huge. Employment status is a core identity in the United States. "What do you do?" is one of the first questions you ask a stranger at a party. The answer is almost always a job description. People who aren't in the workforce sometimes feel compelled to offer an explanation. No one says they are receiving disability benefits. In this country at least, our work defines us. The stakes are high.

Applying for a job requires even more courage for a person who has internalized the stigma of their diagnosis. "They won't hire a crazy person like me. Why bother trying?" Research shows that this type of thinking discourages many people from applying for a job: "Self-stigma seems to be an important internal barrier to seeking employment," even stronger than a person's past experiences of discrimination. A person who has overcome this additional challenge has achieved more than other applicants. They have cleared two hurdles instead of just one. Being hired contradicts the belief that no one would hire them. Part of the payoff is a positive new identity as an "employee." Both the accomplishment of getting a job and the higher status it confers boost self-confidence and may lead to risk-taking in other areas of life.

Christina Fox and Tammy Melvin struggled to hold down jobs due to mental illness. Now they work together at the JBS employment program, helping people in similar situations find and keep jobs. When I asked for a success story, they both wanted to talk first about the same person. He came into the program with a diagnosis of schizophrenia. He wouldn't even talk, let alone participate in any activities. He seemed hopeless. If he didn't believe in himself enough to apply, or wouldn't speak during an interview, his master's degree from a top research university and advanced computer skills wouldn't matter. Tammy described her approach: "I just really bragged on him about the education he had, and you know how you don't get that far and not have a whole lot of knowledge up there, you know." It turns out that was all he needed. He landed a job that pays $75,000 a year.

A high salary is great, but just having a job is what matters most for self-esteem. Christina described an assembly-line position weighing out little packages of nails, putting them into boxes, and sticking on labels. "It gives people that sense of 'Hey, I'm doing something.' It gets them out of the house, you know. And technically, they're working." Tammy explained, "just getting back out and, yeah, being successful. And the camaraderie, the work and, you know, it just helps you mentally so much." Christina and Tammy don't even ask about their clients' diagnoses or medication. Employment is the treatment.

Having an address can be just as therapeutic as having a job. Place defines all of us in fundamental ways. At a party, "Where are you from?" or "Where do you live?" often follows "What do you do?" And it's very hard to host your own party without your own space. And in between parties, relationships are possible only among people who can find one another. It shouldn't be surprising that people with good housing are less lonely. Recall from chapter 6 the Birmingham REACT team client who reconnected with his mother and the client who walks five miles each way, twice a week, to visit his friend and fellow client. Human connection is key to a positive identity.

*　*　*

Some mental health diagnoses carry positive connotations, such as creativity. Along with a bipolar diagnosis, my psychiatrist gave me a copy of the 1993 book by the psychiatrist Kay Redfield Jamison, *Touched with Fire: Manic-Depressive Illness and the Artistic Temperament*. In it, Jamison argues persuasively that bipolar disorder is associated with artistic genius, citing empirical research and scores of historical examples. The relatively high rate of bipolar disorder among extremely creative people is undeniable. People with bipolar disorder can be successful despite the diagnosis, and maybe sometimes even because of it.

Subsequent research regarding the association between bipolar disorder and creativity has been mixed. A 2022 article reviewing recent studies concluded that "it is not possible to say that [bipolar disorder] patients are more creative than healthy controls or than patients with other mental disorders." The authors suggest that Jamison was wrong. But the new studies examine *average* creativity levels, whereas Jamison and the research she cited focused on the rate of bipolar disorder only among extremely creative people. That distinction is critical.

A high percentage of people with bipolar disorder have significant cognitive deficits and other serious symptoms. People in this category would almost certainly do poorly on tests of creativity, which would tend to bring down the bipolar average. Mathematically, there must be a substantial number of people with bipolar disorder who have above-average creativity. How far above average? One possibility is that more than half of people with bipolar disorder are slightly more creative than the average. A more plausible explanation is that a smaller percentage of highly creative people are pulling up the bipolar average. Properly understood, the new studies do not disprove Jamison's claim—if anything, they support it. For better and worse, some people with bipolar disorder are "touched with fire," while many others are burned by it.

The mere existence of high-achieving people with serious mental illness is enough to call into question several negative stereotypes. A psychiatric diagnosis does not always lead to mental incapacity, or even impaired judgment. Some people with mental illness make much better than average decisions. They are famous for their achievements, not infamous for acts of violence. Every human being has multiple identities. No one is just a diagnosis.

Celebrating geniuses (and celebrities, chapter 10) is great, but giving hope matters much more. Even a few success stories prove that people with a serious mental disorder can function as well as people without a diagnosis, and sometimes better. The illness makes some things harder, but not everything. The things you devote yourself to, you can do as well as anyone. You can even be one of the best. That's what my psychiatrist was trying to tell me.

Jamison's 1996 memoir, *An Unquiet Mind: A Memoir of Moods and Madness*, remains a classic, but there are now scores of memoirs written by people with mental illness, especially bipolar disorder. It has become its own genre. Every one of these books is a success story. People experiencing crippling anxiety, full-blown mania, deep depression, or paranoid delusions rarely write books. Van Gogh was a genius, but he did not write a memoir. Books about geniuses are powerful, but behind every memoir is a person who recovered enough to muster the energy and discipline to write a whole book. That's not easy. Writers like Jamison challenge popular negative stereotypes, stereotypes that many people with mental illness come to believe about themselves.

The public is terrified of people with schizophrenia. As discussed in chapter 1, research shows that schizophrenia, unlike other mental illnesses, is in fact associated with a higher risk of violence during psychotic episodes. But the public's fear is not driven by data, or at least not only by data. The perception of dangerousness is heightened by sensational media coverage and portrayals in movies, shows, and online videos. Fear is what leads to avoidance by the public and to the social isolation of people with schizophrenia. The Hearing Voices Network facilitates support groups for "voice hearers" and other people with unusual visions, thoughts, and beliefs. Studies have shown that participation reduces stress, improves self-esteem, and reduces self-stigma. Participants often "go on to build some relationships with the outside world." The voices may not stop, but voice hearers learn how to reframe them in a positive way. "When voice hearers gain a better understanding of their voices, they begin to make the shift from being a passive sufferer to one of being in charge of the voices." The goal is to create an empowered new identity, not simply to manage symptoms. The patient, not the doctor, decides whether a symptom that does not hurt anyone else is good or bad.

Here is a small example. An older man told his doctors about the tiny people he saw all over his house, one in "western garb." As evidence, the man showed the doctors a rock with "teeth marks." "Lilliputian hallucinations" is the medical term for this rare condition. For this and other reasons, the doctors prescribed an antipsychotic medication. When this caused the man to no longer see the little people, he became depressed and anxious. He had lost his friends and was concerned about their well-being. The medication had benefits that probably outweighed the costs. But the important point is that the man considered losing the little people to be a cost, not a benefit.

Recognizing the subjectivity of perception can support positive identity and mitigate self-stigma. The best way to help a person experiencing a nonconsensus reality may not always be to impose a different reality. The overwhelming majority of people with schizophrenia do not act out violently against others any more than the man who saw friendly little people hurt his neighbors. Being told over and over that the voices do not exist may exacerbate rather than comfort the person who hears them.

* * *

To avoid the label "mental patient," some people refuse to accept the diagnosis or refuse treatment. Other people accept the label and treatment. Either way, the diagnosis sets a person apart from others and may lead to feelings of isolation. A person can be alone without being lonely, but there is no substitute for relationships and a community of peers. Intersectionality provides both opportunities and challenges.

The first step toward recovery is asserting oneself. A person with crippling self-doubt cannot take that step. Overcoming that barrier and taking even a very small step is growth. Whatever the outcome, it demonstrates that the person has the ability to make their own decisions and follow through. That the person chooses to use those abilities at all means that they value themself enough to try. Self-worth is a prerequisite for self-advocacy. Advocating for oneself in one area makes it easier to do so in many areas. Self-advocacy is especially important in doctor's offices, clinics, and hospitals. Autonomy in treatment has been shown to reduce self-stigma. One question to a provider often leads to another question, which can create a positive feedback loop. Research shows that self-advocacy improves clinical outcomes.

Self-stigma has many causes. There are the symptoms of the illness itself, of course. But the symptoms are only part of the problem. It is impossible for a person with a diagnosis to ignore pervasive societal stigma. And while our approach to mental illness has changed over time, it remains fractured and dysfunctional. The public doesn't seem to care much about people with serious mental illness. An individual with a mental health diagnosis may feel like less than a person, because they are viewed and treated that way. At least in the United States.

Canada is doing much better. One study found that just 9 percent of Canadians with a serious mental illness had high self-stigma. In the United States, the number was 37 percent. What explains such a massive disparity? It can't be the illness. Symptoms don't care about lines on a map. The rate of serious mental illness may be different in the two countries, but that cannot be the whole explanation either, because only people with a diagnosis answered the question. The huge disparity in self-stigma must be caused in part by differences in how the two countries *respond* to mental illness. In one survey, well over 50 percent of Canadian respondents supported increasing taxes to provide better services for people with schizophrenia. That money would be in addition to the amount Canadian taxpayers already spend on universal healthcare. Canada views healthcare as a human right, which seems to include mental healthcare. But whatever Canada is doing right, the United States should be copying it.

IDENTITY

Having a mental illness is not all bad. The phrase "overcoming self-stigma" suggests that the goal is returning to a prediagnosis sense of self. But why stop there? There is no upper limit on a positive identity. Every person, with or without a mental illness, can always grow. "Building a stronger sense of self" is therefore a more accurate and hopeful framing. In some ways, the negative stereotypes are not just wrong, they are backwards. A person with a mental illness must be stronger than other people to achieve the same level of success. And the people interviewed in this book are better at what they do because of their difficult experiences, not in spite of them.

TAKEAWAYS

- Each of us becomes "a mental patient" the moment we are diagnosed.
- Identities like race, gender, sexuality, and religion complicate mental illness.
- Peer support, employment, and housing are powerful ways to create a positive identity.
- Less obvious ways include music, soccer, and travel (especially to Canada).

CONCLUSION

The mental healthcare system in the United States is a burning building. The people I interviewed for this book escaped long enough to catch their breath, then ran right back into the fire to save others. Their stories are inspiring and instructive, but not exceptional. There is an invisible army of peers working every day to help others succeed in a failing system. Many of these helpers are also policy advocates, demanding systemic reform. None are helpless victims.

Readers may find it difficult to reconcile their negative perceptions about mental illness with the people they encountered in the pages of this book. These are human beings doing their best for one another. Their diagnoses—which range from schizophrenia and bipolar disorder to anorexia, depression, and PTSD—constitute only a small window into their lives. Some have struggled with illegal substance use, some have been involved with the criminal justice system, but none represents a serious danger toward others. In fact, they are doing what they can to help other people with similar struggles. Their stories will probably never make the nightly news or a feature film. In mental health, as in other areas, successes are largely invisible while dramatic failures grab all the attention.

This book has lessons for general readers, for policymakers, and for peers. The stigma attached to serious mental illness is pervasive. Indeed, it would be hard to understand the deep pathologies of our current system if this were not true. It is easy to see the thumbprints of disdain and demonization, from police-led crisis response to criminalization. But a broader and more insidious form of stigma—dehumanization—colors everything. People are reduced to their diagnosis and medications rather than being asked about their own goals.

Focusing solely on mental illness rather than on the complete lived experiences of people with mental illness is myopic. Policymakers too often view the mental healthcare system as consisting of only three levels: crisis, institutionalization, and outpatient medical care (chart 1), as discussed in chapters 1 through 4.

Chart One: The Illness-Oriented Mental Healthcare System

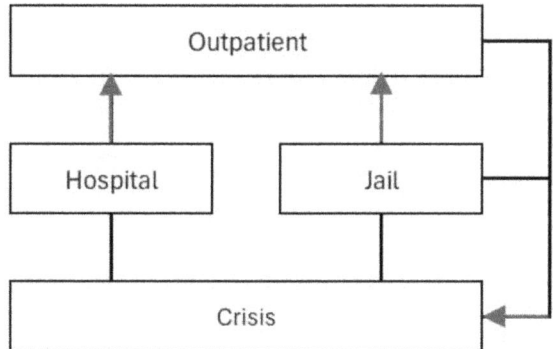

Policymakers often fail to recognize that success with a serious mental illness depends on things like affordable housing and meaningful employment, not just detention and medication. The reforms described in the illness-oriented mental healthcare system will never achieve their full potential without progress in the areas discussed in chapters 5 through 11 (chart 2). It is all connected. It all matters. For example, when people are released from jail or hospital and are unwilling to access outpatient medical care, the prevailing wisdom goes, they fall back into crisis and the cycle repeats. Faced with increasing homelessness or high-profile acts of violence, policymakers criminalize sleeping outside and expand the criteria for involuntary treatment. But a successful life and positive mental health require much more than the right meds—things like adequate housing, a supportive community, education, and employment are essential.

Chart Two: A Whole-Person Mental Healthcare System

```
    [Identity]        [Humanity]         [Advocacy]

         [Education] ↔ [Employment] ----┐
               ↑           ↑            |
              [     Housing     ] ------|
                     ↑                  |
         ┌───→[    Community    ] ------|
         |           ↑                  |
         |    [    Outpatient   ]       |
         |       ↑         ↑            |
         |   [Hospital]  [Jail]         |
         |       ↑         ↑            |
         └───[      Crisis      ]←──────┘
```

Dotted line reflects lower probability of relapse at higher stages of recovery.

This book charts a recovery-oriented, whole-person mental healthcare system, as outlined in chart 2. Starting at the bottom, genuinely dangerous crises will still sometimes lead to hospitalization or even jail, but in many cases, crises can be safely de-escalated at an EmPATH unit, peer respite program, or community crisis center (chapters 1 through 3). Some people cycling through jail or hospital will still need intensive outpatient interventions, like Assertive Community Treatment and Assisted Outpatient Treatment (chapter 4).

But many people can achieve stability without such intensive interventions, provided they have supportive community care (chapter 5) and adequate housing (chapter 6). Employment and education (chapters 7 and 8) are gateways to quality medical care, financial security and, for many, a sense of self-worth. At every stage of recovery, people with mental illness can help one another and themselves by engaging in direct service and advocacy (chapter 9). Long-term, they can work to foster recognition of their shared humanity (chapter 10) and build positive identities (chapter 11).

The similarity between the organization of this book and Maslow's hierarchy of human needs is not coincidental. Psychologist Abraham Maslow developed his theory by examining how successful individuals achieve "self-actualization." Maslow argued that a human being must generally meet basic physical needs, like food and shelter, before tacking intermediate psychological needs, like relationships and esteem, and then finally advancing upward to creative self-fulfillment. Maslow and I define success in the same way: setting and achieving one's own life goals—that's Mike Autrey's definition of "recovery" (introduction).

This is not to deny that mental illness can limit options. And an individual's mental health recovery is only as secure as the weakest link in the chain. Bad luck in any area can precipitate joblessness, homelessness, or a mental health crisis. But crisis and institutionalization are not inevitable, even for individuals with the greatest needs. Some people will require robust wraparound services like those provided by the REACT team in Birmingham, Alabama, which combines housing placement and in-home care (chapter 4). Many other individuals with less severe mental illness or greater social or economic resources can succeed with intensive support in just a few areas. Housing is often the key to accessing other resources in the community, but sometimes employment, educational, or community support is all that an individual needs to achieve independence.

This book highlights existing policies and programs that have been demonstrated to be effective, some of which even pay for themselves. Recall the RAISE-ETP program for first-episode psychosis (chapter 8). Researchers estimate that the program could pay for itself just by avoiding the need for future government benefits for participants. Other intensive short-term programs can decrease total government expenditures over a lifetime. This was almost certainly the case for Samantha Smith (chapter 7). She was able to maintain employment through periods of deep depression because her private health insurance covered an Intensive Outpatient Program. The care offered by this program allowed her to keep her job and health insurance (and pay her taxes) instead of collecting government disability benefits and relying on the public mental healthcare system.

Cost-effective interventions like this are not widely available due to massive workforce shortages, the result of chronic public and private mental health underfunding. In 2024, more than one-third (122 million) of the U.S. population lived in an area with a shortage of mental health professionals. Recognizing the value of lived experience could be a big part of the solution. The mental healthcare system could be turning more patients into peer service providers.

The U.S. Department of Labor does not have an occupational code for peer support specialist. As a result, there are no national statistics about the size or composition of this hidden army. The PEER Support Act would correct that omission (see chapter 9). In addition, the Act would commission a report and recommendations regarding state practices with respect to criminal background checks for peer support specialists. Given the disproportionate impact of the criminal system on people with mental illness, proponents of the Act are concerned that states are disqualifying potential peer support specialists for too many types of low-level offenses. The PEER Support Act would also codify the Office of Recovery and the requirement that it be led by a peer. No more relegation to the coat closet (or exit door) by a new and reactionary presidential administration. We need experienced leaders like Paolo del Vecchio (chapter 9) shaping national policy.

The second Trump administration's extreme defunding agenda across the federal government demonstrates the crucial importance of clear limits on executive power. Of course, Congress would remain free to make deep cuts to programs like Medicaid and Social Security, as it chose to do by approving Trump's budget bill in 2025. But massive changes like this leave open many details of implementation. There will be opportunities to protect high-priority programs. People with lived experience having a seat at the table is essential, whether the budget is $10 billion or $1 billion.

Enforcing existing federal law more aggressively is another way to improve the lives of people with mental illness. The ADA and the Rehabilitation Act already prohibit discrimination based on mental disability in crisis response, involuntary detention, prison conditions, employment, and education. These laws are woefully underenforced. The Department of Justice already has the authority to bring ADA challenges against state and local authorities. It could be doing more to support lawsuits against private employers and educational institutions. No doubt many businesses and schools are trying to adhere to the law, but many others must be taught that discrimination is not only wrong, but it can hurt their financial bottom line. It is not fair to put all the cost and risk of litigating antidiscrimination cases on the injured parties, who by definition are already dealing with mental health challenges.

Sometimes, the same policies and decisions that are negatively affecting people with mental illness are hurting other employees as well. People with mental illness can be the proverbial canaries in the coal mine. More flexible work hours, better leave policies, and narrower conduct codes (chapter 7) can make an employer more attractive to all applicants and improve retention across the board. Why not accommodate reasonable employee requests? Remote work during and after the pandemic is an example of what flexibility looks like. Of course, employers can demand in-person work, but they must now consider whether that demand will lead productive employees to quit. No-questions-asked "mental health days" are another example.

This book has additional implications for people living with mental illness. The stories show that successful recovery in the face of overwhelming obstacles is possible. Hopefully, the stories will also inspire service and advocacy. With mental and socioeconomic stability comes the opportunity for people with SMI to provide direct services to other people with mental illness and to become advocates for them. Disclosure of one's own diagnosis is not required for either role, but it can foster trust and build credibility. Attending a peer-led support group is a powerful way to help oneself and the other participants. Tens of thousands of peers do this every week. Direct service and advocacy often overlap, but need not. Either way, advocacy can and should include seats at the table for people with mental illness. Recall Washington state's "Nothing About Us Without Us" Act (chapter 9), which mandates peer representation on government task forces.

It is not fair to ask people with lived experience to fix the broken mental healthcare system. No one should be expected to run back into a burning building. But the people who have experienced the fire may be the only ones who can lead us to a mental healthcare system that works for the people it is intended to serve. Peers have much to teach and much to give. Peers can connect to and empower one another in ways that non-peers cannot. And many people with serious mental illness *want* to help work for a better system. Listening to their stories is the first step toward more effective and humane policies for people with mental illness and, ultimately, a more just and equitable society.

EPILOGUE

While writing this book, I had my first full-blown manic episode in eighteen years. I know bipolar disorder is a chronic illness, but I had really thought I was in the clear as to the high end of the mood spectrum. I had been stable on lithium for almost two decades. Sure, there were depressive episodes and drug side effects, but I thought keeping up with my meds and sticking to my routine would be enough to stay out of the hospital. Wishful thinking, it turns out.

Friend no more, the lithium had started to impair my kidney function, so my doctors and I decided that I had to add a replacement mood stabilizer, then wean myself off the lithium. That went fine until I was at the smallest dose of lithium, when I spiraled quickly into delusional psychosis. I spent two weeks in an inpatient psychiatric unit, and it took about two months after discharge for my mind to function well enough to make any progress on this book.

One minute I'm writing a book about other people succeeding with mental illness; the next minute I'm back in my own mental health crisis. Before the hospitalization, I was outlining the last chapter. I had too many ideas to squeeze in, which may have been partially the product of hypomania. Or maybe excitement about the book taking shape was cause rather than effect. Causation with mood disorders is often murky. Either way, my notes from this time period are disorganized and unhelpful.

After being forced to take all that time off from writing the book, I decided to go back through the earlier chapters to remind myself of what was in them. I could barely stomach the first two chapters, "Crisis" and "Hospital." My own new traumatic experiences were way too fresh in my mind. It was easier to revise the "Jail" chapter because, once again, I avoided the criminal system by agreeing to go voluntarily to the hospital before the mania spiraled and the police were called. My wife Caroline deserves all the credit by intervening at exactly the right moment. That choice probably also meant I kept my job and got sick leave rather than getting fired. After hospital discharge, my advantages in the other domains—outpatient care, housing, and education—continued to prop up my recovery. I was discharged to a safe home, supportive family, and ready team of outpatient providers. I went to work on Donna's Law advocacy before I was able to go back to work on this book. I found purpose again before I found focus.

Once again, I had avoided the worst of our broken mental healthcare system due to luck and privilege. Still, this episode underscored for me a few of the major themes of this book. Recovery is not linear, and there is no endpoint. It's amazing how you can have every advantage—every single advantage—and one small thing, one breeze near your house of cards, and the whole thing collapses. It doesn't matter how big your house of cards was, how sturdy it used to be; it just collapses in the same way for everybody who has the same illness. We all have the potential to go to exactly the same place: complete and uncontrolled crisis. The people with mental illness in this book working on behalf of others know this. Success is always provisional. Those who run back into the fire risk being burned just like the people they are trying to save.

I unpacked the significance of my most recent hospitalization and its other connections to this book in stages. I started the process with my own memories and through conversations with Caroline. She delayed taking me to the hospital as long as she could. She hoped she'd be able to quell my increasingly grandiose delusions with extra meds we stockpiled for this situation. In the middle of a sleepless night, I ran back and forth in our bedroom. The tipping point was when my paranoia started to include Caroline and I resisted the meds she was offering to help me sleep. "Put them by the side of the bed and I'll decide whether to take them later." We have always agreed that resisting reasonable meds is the trigger for hospitalization. That next morning, she explained to our kids why I might not be home in the evening and made sure I said goodbye.

Both aware of my diagnosis from young ages, they took it in stride, or at least without question.

Caroline asked a neighbor to drive us to the hospital because she thought I might grab the steering wheel on the way. I offered plenty of unneeded driving advice from the back seat, but didn't put up any physical resistance. I didn't want to be in the emergency department, but didn't try to leave. Caroline was prepared, at one point producing two peanut butter sandwiches from ziplock bags. As a doctor, she sends people to that emergency room all the time and you just never know how long you'll be waiting. Then they whisked me away and abruptly told her to leave. Families were not allowed, they said. Caroline was upset about that and more upset about me being sick again. She was crying and had to be picked up.

They called Caroline about an hour later saying I would be admitted; they were waiting for a bed, and she could come back to wait with me. She found me "scared and stressed" without her in the loud and crowded emergency room. I called out that the man on a gurney next to me was dying. I do remember thinking that because of a blank line on his heart monitor. The woman sitting with him was "very unhappy" with me (Caroline's words). Being in the ER is stressful enough without a crazy neighbor yelling that a loved one is dying. Eventually, the special psychiatric waiting room opened up. It was single-occupancy and quiet, with a door that closed and blue rubbery furniture.

A bed became available that afternoon. Two staff members wheeled me upstairs to the door of the locked unit. Caroline asked the "angry guy" at the door what happened next.

> Staff: You go.
> Caroline: When can I come and visit normally? I spend as much time as I can with him when he's in the hospital.
> Staff: Well, you can't do that here. . . . The policy on this unit is no visitors for two weeks.
> Caroline: That's ridiculous. Why?
> Staff: So that we can assess the patients and observe them.
> Caroline: We already know the diagnosis, so like, we're not trying to make a diagnosis here.
> Staff: Well, that's our policy.

And then he shut the door in her face.

On the other side of that door, my third hospitalization would be orders of magnitude more traumatizing than my first two. I came out of the hospital furious, primarily about being put in seclusion. That episode was the focus of a trauma journaling exercise I did a couple of months after my release. Here are some excerpts:

> *They put me in a box: one door, padded, along with the walls and floor. Nothing else. I pleaded to no avail. I tried everything I could think of to get out, and I could think of a lot of crazy stuff to try in my still manic and agitated state. . . . I held my plastic bracelet in the window on the door, while simultaneously pushing out the bottom of my robe under the door. Why that would work I can't remember. Creativity points? The soft spot did not conceal a secret lever either. I cannot remember events leading up to my imprisonment, nor the duration—I only have bright white flashes of being thrown in and trying to get out. I don't remember any explanation for why I was being put into seclusion or any indication as to whether and how I might get out. I believed I was being put in there to die, alone.*

Seclusion eventually ended, though I have no memory of that. Indeed, my lack of memory became another source of trauma. Again from my post-hospitalization journal:

> *One of the most traumatic moments was when I finally had enough mental capacity to figure out how long I had been on the unit. Maybe I stole art supplies, but I drew a calendar and counted out five or so days. I couldn't believe that this time was stolen from me. My memories covered only a few moments. If they had told me I had been there one day I would have believed them. I imagine it's easier for staff to restrain, sedate, and isolate patients believing that the patients won't remember and might even come to thank them later. But we don't always forget, and I bet some of what we do forget has lingering unconscious impacts. Staff and patients probably agree that seclusion and restraint are "last resorts," but the question is what else must be*

tried first, second, and third. I don't know how disruptive and/or confrontational my behavior was, but being put in seclusion days in a row is a helluva lot.

By the time I wrote this last entry, I had peeked at my online medical record, which included multiple entries about seclusion. Something else popped out:

"Restraint chair." What the hell is that? I have no memory of being restrained in a chair, but it's in my medical notes. Is it used to hold a patient still while they receive an injection of sedatives? Longer? I don't remember any injections either, but the chart is filled with references to meds. Seeing this in the notes raises complicated reactions. They did try other things before isolation, it seems. The notes also detail disruptive behavior. Maybe the forced meds and restraint and isolation were necessary "last resorts" and I have nothing to complain about. . . . But blame is beside the point really. The issue now is trauma, which doesn't depend on cause or blame. It just is. This moment, really [a] period of days, when my mind failed almost completely and I was treated like less than a person. I remember, assholes!

I needed more information than was available in the online portal, so I requested my complete medical records. The first ninety-three pages detail my inpatient stay. The staff put me into a seclusion room at least four days in a row. These days blur together so much that I would have believed it if the medical record indicated only one time in seclusion. I believed the staff was trying to kill me. I believed I was going to die in that room. I remember screaming nonstop, trying passwords and gestures I thought might have a chance of getting me out. From a staff note: "Over an hour later and patient continues to press on seclusion door, speak in delusional statements, disorganized, and tangential." Clinical language for existential terror. For me, seclusion was torture.

Most of the first week is a blur, but eventually my mind started to clear with time and a new combination of meds. As I was approaching discharge, I asked one of the attendants why I had been put in the seclusion room and whether I had been violent. "Not toward me," the staff member replied. At the time he said this, I thought to myself, "then why the hell was I restrained?" I was deaf to the implication that I may have been violent toward others. And the records do indicate that I was physically and verbally abusive with other staff. Did I resist seclusion in particular? Apparently not. According to the attendant, I just went limp when they grabbed my arms. In my first two hospitalizations in Chicago, by contrast, I remember my disruptive behavior resulting in forced medication—sometimes called "chemical restraints." That was humiliating and disorienting, but nothing compared to my time in seclusion. In Chicago, I even developed a special affection for the large male nurse, Andy, who held me down while the drugs were being administered.

It is tempting to conclude that the staff during my most recent hospitalization should have at least relied on forced medication instead of seclusion as a less traumatizing alternative. Even with the benefit of hindsight, however, I can't say that for sure, for several reasons. First, they *did* attempt to address my threatening behavior with sedating medication. My medical record is replete with references to such meds: "Had 2 episodes of agitation yesterday requiring PRN medications for agitation, but no seclusion." For me, it seems, the drugs were not enough. The staff resorted to seclusion after physical outbursts. And when seclusion failed, the hospital suspended the protocol and used even more sedating medications. I was very, very sick. There were no good solutions.

Two nights in a row I was put into the "restraint chair." As noted, I have no memory of this, which I consider now to be a great mercy. Did it match the trauma of seclusion? Exceed it? The photo I found on the internet does not answer these questions, though the chair looks well-padded and reasonably ergonomic. I hope the straps are tight enough to eliminate any false hope of escape. Otherwise, a person in distress might fight against confinement just as I fought against seclusion. Tight straps would also seem to reduce the chances of injury—less bruising if you can't build up limb speed as you flail.

Why was this hospitalization so much worse? One possibility is that the symptoms were worse. There is clearly some truth in that. Near the end of my stay, a staff member wrote: "He said that he had been hospitalized three times, but this time he was more confused and it sucks being confused." I confessed to staff at least once that I couldn't remember why I had been put into seclusion, which obviously made the experience more terrifying. I pounded against the door when sitting quietly was the way out. But I don't think the greater intensity of the mania alone can explain the difference. Something about the Alabama unit exacerbated the trauma of hospitalization. My searing memory of seclusion stands out, but ultimately I don't think this use of force, or forced treatment generally, is a sufficient explanation. Greater use of force caused more trauma, to be sure, but perhaps greater use of force was necessitated by something else: a failure of trust.

* * *

The primary goal of inpatient hospitalization these days is to find a combination of prescriptions to stabilize patients enough to discharge them. My medical record appears to confirm this. The reason for the admission was "safety and medication management." There was no individual or group therapy mentioned in the doctor's note, only "milieu activities." Those activities were mentioned once in the online medical record. I remember just one art class.

But the full ninety-three-page medical record tells a different story. Here are some of the things I don't remember: daily group activities that my condition prevented me from participating in; daily social worker interactions that I usually blew off; spitting out meds; screaming random names and numbers while others were watching television; touching other patients or their possessions; escape attempts; running up and down hallways; and verbal and physical abuse of staff that I blanch at reading now. I even used the "N" word. My righteous indignation at neglect and mistreatment by the inpatient staff is deflated like a balloon. I really don't know how to feel. Now who's the asshole?

Given my impaired memory, I cannot criticize the hospital for its use of force. All of it may have been justified. On one occasion, after cursing at staff, they administered a formal violence risk assessment before administering medication for agitation and putting me into the restraint chair. Force did not work well, however: "Patient continues to be verbally aggressive while in restraints cursing and making demands. It appears that him being 1:1 while in restraints made him more agitated." Perhaps that experience was part of the reason for the use of seclusion the next day. That didn't go well either: "[Patient] with psychomotor agitation for the entirety of the seclusion period." I think that must have been the period of seclusion I remember and the worst thing that has ever happened to me. Using force at this point was arguably necessary for the safety of the other patients and staff even though it felt like torture for me. But what went wrong to get to this point?

Maybe it started at admission when they sent Caroline away—the one person I trusted completely. The hospital would later cite privacy concerns, even though I came to the hospital voluntarily with my wife and cutting off all connections to the outside world was deeply damaging to me. Furthermore, under federal law, providers are allowed to share information even when the patient is unable to meaningfully consent or object, if providers conclude that sharing is in the "best interests" of the patient, which it would have been in my case.

A couple of examples: One of my first days on the unit, the psychiatrist told me he was ordering a head CT scan. The note records my reply as "Oh wonderful . . . would Caroline [wife] want that to happen?" It was clear from the beginning whom I trusted with my medical decisions. I told my medical team directly that there was a "trust issue." The treatment team visit one day "ended abruptly" when I stated that I did "not trust anyone and wanted everyone to leave." There was one person I trusted, and she was not there.

About midway through the hospitalization, a nurse's note described me as "confrontational today, stating that 'y'all want to keep me here in prison,' 'I know you don't want my wife to visit me'—in response to me telling him that I was excited his wife was going to get to visit him today. He isn't redirectable for questioning." It went better the following day. The attending psychiatrist understood and arranged for a visit with Caroline when I was agitated: "[Patient] was calmer after visitation." Of course, a spousal visit or even phone call may not have been feasible during every moment of crisis.

Epilogue

There was another reason Caroline didn't push harder to visit sooner, which I learned only months later when I sat down to interview her: More than once during that first week, I refused to speak with her on the phone. "I knew you were still sick because you weren't even asking to call. And so I called. You know, I would call all the time." Sometimes, the nurse who answered would ask Caroline to try to convince me to take my meds. "And he's like . . . ." Caroline shifts to the third person in the middle of our conversation. "Do you hear? I just said 'he's like,' because it was not you, you know, it was like a different person." I'd ask Caroline whether to take the meds, but I'd sometimes hang up before she could answer, and another time I just said "bullshit." And more than once I told her not to come visit.

The new doctor who finally gave permission for Caroline to visit thought it could be good for me and would lower my "stress level." I thought I remembered what happened during those visits, but Caroline filled in some embarrassing details. I pulled an emergency call string, notwithstanding her instruction not to, multiple times. The staff just glanced over because they knew what I was up to, Caroline observed. I always had a sitter with me. "To make sure you were safe," Caroline said. "And to protect you," I added. "No, I don't think so," she added, they were always there, because "you were in everybody's business, definitely." Caroline's visits were my lifeline back to sanity, just as they had been in Chicago. Whatever else is true, the no-visitor policy in Birmingham made everything worse. Caroline recalls: "Over and over again, every day I was like, 'I'm sure he will be better if I can be with him.' And you know, they're like, 'Oh, no, we've got it under control. It's fine.'" It was not fine.

* * *

It took months for me to recover enough to understand some of the many ways my hospitalization experience connected to this book. The most important thing I take away now is the critical importance of peer participation in decision-making, from crisis response all the way through policy-making. If the patient perspective is not represented, it will not be given adequate weight. Ideally, there would be somebody in the room who has been tied down to that restraint chair and understands how that feels to decide, "Okay, now it's really necessary." In an inpatient psychiatric unit, that will often be impractical in the moment, but staff protocols can and should reflect patient experiences collected after the fact.

But we can do better than improving general protocols—we can better tailor interventions to individual patient preferences, even if they are in crisis and lack decision-making capacity. People ought to be allowed to express their preferences in advance and have those preferences respected to the fullest extent possible, especially people who have been hospitalized before. This is no different in principle than advance directives and living wills for end-of-life decision-making. Indeed, many states specifically authorize psychiatric advance directives (PADs), which are designed precisely for this purpose. For example, one model PAD form includes a long checklist of preferred options for inpatient emergency interventions such as "time out/privacy," "show of authority/force," and "shift my attention to something else." Should the selected options fail or be infeasible, the form provides for a rank ordering of chemical restraints, physical restraints, and seclusion. Seclusion would be last on my list. On the flip side, I would request and consent in my PAD to as many visits by Caroline as possible.

What happens in inpatient psych units is important in its own right, but the implication is much broader than that. People with lived experience need to be in every room, or decisions will systematically undervalue their perspectives. "Nothing about us without us" is much more than a slogan. When making policy decisions—like how much to invest in affordable housing or in treatment programs for first-episode psychosis or in any policy promoting the recovery of people with mental illness—we need to ask: "Are the people with lived experience part of that conversation?" And if not, we will underinvest in these programs every time, because the decision-makers don't know what the final fallback option—forced treatment—feels like. The true cost of force is known only to those who have felt it. Everyone agrees in theory that force is a last resort; the issue is what else must be tried before using it.

The subjective experience of survivors is not the only consideration, but it is the most important one, and the least well represented. And what is true for forced treatment is true for every other good and bad outcome discussed in this book, from career success to homelessness: Only those with experience know how it feels. Each peer should have the power to decide what recovery means to them individually. We need to be involved not just in direct support, but in program design and funding decisions as well. This book captures only a few of our voices. Every voice matters.

ACKNOWLEDGMENTS

This book is dedicated to the memory of Kathleen O'Grady, who helped me believe in myself and my story enough to write it. I heard an echo of Kathleen's voice at the end of one interview. When I told the woman I thought her inspiring story would make a much better book than mine, she replied without hesitation: "Thank you for being willing to share your experiences too. It all matters."

I cannot thank enough the amazing people who shared their stories with me: Mike Autrey, TJ Bradley, Alex Brass, Jon Brock, Amy Brinkley, Joyce Campbell, Leslie Carpenter, Delores Cimini, Christi Collins, Paolo del Vecchio, Maurice "Moe" Egan, Anita Fisher, Anna Fiscus-Surita, Christina Fox, Ethan Frost, Amy Griesel, Duncan Gibson, Rick Gish, Jennifer Harrell, Marie Holliday, Tom Hopkins, Evelyn Graham-Nyaasi, Jim Gottstein, Stephanie Lyn Kaufman-Mthimkhulu, Sonny Leppala, Jesse Mangan, Ann Marshall, Thomson McKorkle, Tammy Melvin, Vania Mendoza, Faith Myers, Robbie Myrick, Leslie Napper, Cyrus Napolitano, Stephanie Nieves, Charisse Parker, Shannon Pagdon, Hector Ramirez, Mark Richards, Marilyn Roberts, Rafael Rodriguez, Harvey Rosenthal, Kathy Sawyer, Eric Smith, Samantha Smith, Steve Stone, Laura Van Tosh, Justin Volpe, Melissa Wettengel, and Scott Zeller.

Several other people were essential. My former professor, mentor, serial coauthor, and friend, Ian Ayres, provided outstanding feedback and constant encouragement. James Tucker jumpstarted the process with introductions to a dozen experts in the field. My "book buddy," Chad Topaz, kept my spirits up during the difficult early stages. Brad Snyder and David Lat shared their book-publishing wisdom. David Patton gave

Acknowledgments

helpful comments on chapter 3. The General Writers—John and Alecia Archibald, Daniel Brow, Jonathan Weisen, and Natasha Zaretsky—improved the book substantially and helped me get it over the finish line. My virtual writing partner, Yusi Wang, provided critical accountability and camaraderie. I could not have asked for a better agent than Gary Heidt, or a better editor than Jake Bonar.

My colleagues at the University of Alabama School of Law, including Deans Mark Brandon and Bill Brewbaker, were unfailingly supportive and helpful. Daiquiri Steele provided helpful feedback on chapter 7. Thanks also to the Bounds Law Library staff and my outstanding student collaborators: Kamryn Carpenter, Alex Landgraf, Courtney Lekai, Greg Martin, Mary Kathryn Morgan, and John Pace. Alex in particular provided outstanding editorial feedback on the entire manuscript.

Boundless gratitude for the unwavering love of my parents, Charles and Freda, and my brothers, Ray and John. Finally, in order of appearance in my life, Caroline, Adam, and Charlotte not only make this book possible, they make everything possible. I love you.

NOTES

INTRODUCTION

vii "Less than half . . ." Substance Abuse and Mental Health Services Administration, *Key Substance Use and Mental Health Indicators in the United States: Results from the 2021 National Survey on Drug Use and Health*, HHS Publication No. PEP22-07-01-005, NSDUH Series H-57 (Center for Behavioral Health Statistics and Quality and Substance Abuse and Mental Health Services Administration, 2022), https://www.samhsa.gov/data/report/2021-nsduh-annual-national-report.

vii "Over a million . . ." Lorna Collier, "Incarceration Nation," *American Psychological Association* 45, no. 9 (2014), https://www.apa.org/monitor/2014/10/incarceration.

vii "One study counted . . . over half a million people in 2006." Ingrid D. Goldstrom, Jean Campbell, Joseph A. Rogers, David B. Lambert, Beatrice Blacklow, Marilyn J. Henderson, and Ronald W. Manderscheid, "National Estimates for Mental Health Mutual Support Groups, Self-Help Organizations, and Consumer-Operated Services," *Administration and Policy in Mental Health and Mental Services Research* 33, no. 1 (2006): 92–103, https://doi.org/10.1007/s10488-005-0019-x.

CHAPTER 1

3 "Brandon Marshall . . ." Bresaz v. County of Santa Clara, 136 F. Supp. 3d 1125 (N.D. Cal. 2015).

3 "Marshall was a forty-three-year-old . . . degree in computer science." Scott Herhold, "Herhold: The Strange, Sad History of Brandon Marshall," SiliconValley.com, updated August 17, 2016, https://www.siliconvalley.com/2014/09/11/herhold-the-strange-sad-history-of-brandon-marshall/.

3 "Marshall also . . . job mobility and wages." Consolidated Amended Complaint, *In re High-Tech Emp. Antitrust Litig.*, No. 11-CV-2509-LHK (N.D. Cal. Sept. 13, 2011), 2011 WL 11683784.

3 "The case would eventually settle . . ." Settlement Agreement, *In re High-Tech Emp. Antitrust Litig.*, No. 5:11CV02509 (N.D. Cal. Sept. 21, 2013), 2013 WL 8480300.

4 "According to the police . . ." "Mapping Police Violence," Campaign Zero, updated May 5, 2025, https://mappingpoliceviolence.org/.

4 "It has been estimated . . ." Doris A. Fuller, Richard Lamb, Michael Biasotti, and John Snook, *Overlooked in the Undercounted: The Role of Mental Illness in Fatal Law*

Enforcement Encounters (Treatment Advocacy Center Office of Research & Public Affairs, 2015), 1, https://www.tac.org/reports_publications/overlooked-in-the-undercounted-the-role-of-mental-illness-in-fatal-law-enforcement-encounters/.

4 "according to the FBI . . ." "Law Enforcement Officers Killed and Assaulted (LEOKA)," Federal Bureau of Investigation: Uniform Crime Reporting, accessed June 4, 2025, https://ucr.fbi.gov/leoka.

5 "people experiencing a first episode . . ." Sarah Youn, Belinda L. Guadagno, Linda K. Byrne, Amity E. Watson, Sean Murrihy, and Sue M. Cotton, "Systematic Review and Meta-Analysis: Rates of Violence During First-Episode Psychosis (FEP)," *Schizophrenia Bulletin* 50, no. 4 (2024): 757, https://doi.org/10.1093/schbul/sbae010.

5 "Schizophrenia is associated with . . ." Youn et al., "Systematic Review and Meta-Analysis," 757.

5 "The landmark MacArthur study . . . people with mental illness." John Monahan, Henry J. Steadman, Eric Silver, Paul S. Appelbaum, Pamela Clark Robbins, Edward P. Mulvey, Loren Roth, Thomas Grisso, and Steven Banks, *Rethinking Risk Assessment: The MacArthur Study of Mental Disorder and Violence* (Oxford University Press, 2001), 56.

5 "When the effect of living . . . addicted to substances." Henry J. Steadman, Edward P. Mulvey, John Monahan, Pamela Clark Robbins, Paul S. Appelbaum, Thomas Grisso, Loren Roth, and Eric Silver, "Violence by People Discharged from Acute Psychiatric Inpatient Facilities and by Others in the Same Neighborhoods," *Archives of General Psychiatry* 55, no. 5 (1998): 393, doi:10.1001/archpsyc.55.5.393.

6 "Deadly force is allowed . . ." Tennessee v. Garner, 471 U.S. 1, 3 (1985).

6 "A 2024 article . . . resulted in 'serious injury.'" Youn et al., "Systematic Review and Meta-Analysis," 757, 762, 764.

9 "Overall call volume . . . over the phone." Heather Saunders, "988 Suicide & Crisis Lifeline: Two Years After Launch," KFF, July 29, 2024, https://www.kff.org/mental-health/issue-brief/988-suicide-crisis-lifeline-two-years-after-launch/.

9 "The trailblazing CAHOOTS . . . mental health calls." Ben Adam Climer and Brenton Gicker, "CAHOOTS: A Model for Prehospital Mental Health Crisis Intervention," *Psychiatric Times* 38, no. 1 (2021), https://www.psychiatrictimes.com/view/cahoots-model-prehospital-mental-health-crisis-intervention.

9 "approximately 2 percent." Eugene Police Department Crime Analysis Unit, *CAHOOTS Program Analysis 2021 Update* (updated 2022), 5, https://www.eugene-or.gov/DocumentCenter/View/66051/CAHOOTS-program-analysis-2021-update.

9 "75 percent of responders . . ." "Peer-Led Mobile Crisis Response: How It Works," A Greenfield People's Budget, June 2021, https://peoplesbudgetgreenfield.com/cahoots/.

9 "In San Francisco . . ." City and County of San Francisco Street Crisis Response Team, *January 2025 SCRT Report* (2025), 1, https://media.api.sf.gov/documents/Jan_2025_SCRT_Report.pdf.

10 "Savings in a single year . . ." "What Is CAHOOTS?," White Bird Clinic, October 29, 2020, https://whitebirdclinic.org/what-is-cahoots/.

11 "Oklahoma pioneered . . . more than 90 percent." Editorial Board, "The Solution to America's Mental Health Crisis Already Exists," *New York Times*, October 4, 2022, https://www.nytimes.com/2022/10/04/opinion/us-mental-health-community-centers.html.

12 "In Maricopa County . . ." Margaret E. Balfour, Arlene Hahn Stephenson, Ayesha Delany-Brumsey, Jason Winsky, and Matthew L. Goldman, "Cops, Clinicians, or Both? Collaborative Approaches to Responding to Behavioral health Emergencies," *Psychiatric Services* 73, no. 6 (2021): 663, https://psychiatryonline.org/doi/10.1176/appi.ps.202000721.

12 "According to a *Washington Post* database . . ." "Police Shootings Database 2015-2024: Search By Race, Age, Department," *Washington Post*, accessed June 4, 2025, https://www.washingtonpost.com/graphics/investigations/police-shootings-database/.

12 "That's what happened . . ." U.S. Department of Justice Civils Rights Division and U.S. Attorney's Office Northern District of Illinois, *Investigation of the Chicago Police Department* (2017), 37, https://www.justice.gov/d9/chicago_findings_1-13-17.pdf.

13 "Almost exactly ten years . . . fallen to the ground." "16 Shots: The Murder Trial of Jason Van Dyke," CBS News (Chicago), August 30, 2018, https://www.cbsnews.com/chicago/news/16-shots-the-murder-trial-of-jason-van-dyke/.

13 "The department has made progress . . ." "Consent Decree Compliance Dashboard," Chicago Police Department, accessed June 5, 2025, https://www.chicagopolice.org/statistics-data/data-dashboards/consent-decree-compliance-dashboard/.

13 "The overwhelming majority . . ." Youn et al., "Systematic Review and Meta-Analysis," 757.

16 "In 2021, the *New York Times* . . . 'contempt of cop.'" David D. Kirkpatrick, Steve Eder, Kim Barker, and Julie Tate, "Why Many Police Traffic Stops Turn Deadly," *New York Times*, updated November 30, 2021, https://www.nytimes.com/2021/10/31/us/police-traffic-stops-killings.html.

16 "Less than two years . . . beat Nichols to death." Robin Stein, Alexander Cardia, and Natalie Reneau, "71 Commands in 13 Minutes: Officers Gave Tyre Nichols Impossible Orders," *New York Times*, February 1, 2023, https://www.nytimes.com/2023/01/29/us/tyre-nichols-video-assault-cops.html.

CHAPTER 2

18 "The Alabama Insane Hospital . . . in the community." Bill Weaver, "Bryce Hospital (Alabama Insane Hospital)," *Encyclopedia of Alabama*, June 5, 2008, https://encyclopediaofalabama.org/article/bryce-hospital-alabama-insane-hospital/.

19 "The third issue reported . . . double its rated capacity." *The Bryce News: Of the Patients, By the Patients, For the Patients* 1, no. 3 (April 1951): 1.

19 "One journalist described . . . electroshock therapy and solitary confinement." Clifton Slaten, "The 1995 Wyatt Litigation: Beginnings, Trial Strategies, and Results," *Law & Psychology Review* 35 (2011): 179.

Notes

19 "In 1970 . . ." Wyatt v. Stickney, 344 F. Supp. 373, 374 (M.D. Ala. 1972), *aff'd sub nom.* Wyatt v. Aderholt, 503 F.2d 1305 (5th Cir. 1974).
19 "The next year, federal judge Frank Johnson . . ." Wyatt v. Stickney, 325 F. Supp. 781, 785 (M.D. Ala. 1971).
20 "The state initially agreed . . ." *Wyatt*, 344 F. Supp. at 383.
20 "Almost immediately, however . . ." *Aderholt*, 503 F.2d at 1307.
20 "In the end, it took thirty-three years . . ." Wyatt *ex rel.* Rawlins v. Sawyer, 219 F.R.D. 529, 535 (M.D. Ala. 2004).
20 "The state's primary strategy . . ." Weaver, "Bryce Hospital."
20 "Nationwide . . . numbers are unknown." Ted Lutterman, *Trends in Psychiatric Inpatient Capacity, United States and Each State, 1970 to 2018*, Technical Assistance Collaborative Paper, no. 2 (National Association of State Mental Health Program Directors, September 2022), https://robwipond.com/wp-content/uploads/2025/02/Trends-in-Psychiatric-Inpatient-Capacity_United-States-_1970-2018_NASMHPD-2.pdf.
20 "For example, in North Carolina . . ." Dana Miller Ervin, host, *Fractured* (podcast), part 5, "The Mental Health Crisis in North Carolina's Emergency Rooms," WFAE 90.7, May 3, 2024, https://www.wfae.org/podcast/fractured/2024-05-03/the-mental-health-crisis-in-north-carolinas-emergency-rooms.
21 "'The ER is a bright . . ." Ervin, *Fractured*, part 5.
21 "In a 2018 lawsuit . . ." Second Amended Complaint at 14, 34, Doe v. Weaver, 725 F. Supp. 3d 132 (D.N.H. 2024) (No. 18-cv-1039-LM).
21 "In December 2024 . . ." Jon Schoenheider, "For 1st Time Five Years, No Adults Waiting for Inpatient Psychiatric Care in NH Emergency Departments," WMUR, December 6, 2024, https://www.wmur.com/article/inpatient-psychiatric-care-nh-emergency-department/63120039.
22 "Nationally, emergency departments . . ." Loredana Santo, Zachary J. Peters, and Carol J. DeFrances, "Emergency Department Visits Among Adults With Mental Health Disorders: United States, 2017–2019," *NCHS Data Brief* no. 426, December 2021.
22 "One Minneapolis EmPATH unit . . ." "Innovative Emergency Mental Health Treatment Model Takes Off in the Midwest," Medical Alley, April 5, 2023, https://medicalalley.org/innovative-emergency-mental-health-treatment-model-takes-off-in-the-midwest/.
22 "The most important goal . . ." James Lockwood, "EmPATH Units: Improving Psychiatric Emergency Care," BWBR, October 13, 2020, https://www.bwbr.com/2020/10/13/empath-units-improving-psychiatric-emergency-care/.
23 "In 1989 . . ." New York State Office of Mental Health, *2012 Annual Report to the Governor and Legislature of New York State on Comprehensive Psychiatric Emergency Programs*, accessed May 29, 2025, https://omh.ny.gov/omhweb/statistics/cpep_annual_report/2012.pdf.
23 "Alabama since 2020 . . . specialists on staff." Margaret Kates, "Crisis Centers and Clinics: New Mental Health Care Models Attempt to Fill Gaps in Alabama System," AL.com, October 5, 2022, https://www.al.com/news/2022/10/crisis-centers

-and-clinics-new-mental-health-care-models-attempt-to-fill-gaps-in-alabama-system.html.
23 "A pilot study in Utah . . . costs went down." Arlene Hahn Stephenson, Tom Betlach, and Debra A. Pinals, "Innovation and Determination: How Three States Are Achieving Comprehensive, Coordinated, and Sustainable Behavioral Health Crisis Systems," in *From Crisis to Care: Building from 988 and Beyond for Better Mental Health Outcomes*, ed. Debra A. Pinals and Elizabeth S. Hancq (National Association of State Mental Health Program Directors, September 2022), 203, https://library.samhsa.gov/sites/default/files/pep22-01-03-001.pdf.
25 "I WAS MYSELF . . ." Harry R. London, "I Was Myself," *The Bryce News: Of the Patients, By the Patients, For the Patients* 1, no. 3 (April 1951): 2.
25 "In 1974 . . . after this opinion." Jack Drake, "Drafting the Case: The Parallel Legacies of *Wyatt v. Stickney* and *Lynch v. Baxley*," *Law & Psychology Review* 35 (2011): 169–70, 174.
27 "It is estimated that approximately 40 percent . . ." Estina E. Thompson, Harold W. Neighbors, Cheryl Munday, and Steve Trierweiler, "Length of Stay, Referral to Aftercare, and Rehospitalization Among Psychiatric Inpatients," *Psychiatric Services* 54, no. 9 (2003): 1271, https://doi.org/10.1176/appi.ps.54.9.1271.
27 "The legal and ethical questions . . ." See, for example, Graham Danzer and Asha Wilkus-Stone, "The Give and Take of Freedom: The Role of Involuntary Hospitalization and Treatment in Recovery from Mental Illness," *Bulletin of the Menninger Clinic* 79, no. 3 (2015): 255–80, https://doi.org/10.1521/bumc.2015.79.3.255.
28 "Evidence from a long-standing . . ." "NYAPRS Peer Bridger™ Program," Alliance for Rights and Recovery, accessed May 29, 2025, https://rightsandrecovery.org/nyaprs-peer-bridger-program/.
31 "The first episode of the podcast . . ." Jesse Mangan, host, *Committable* (podcast), season 1, episode 1, "Section 12," Podbean, March 17, 2021, https://committablethepodcast.podbean.com/e/s1-episode-1-section-12/.
32 "Civil commitment . . . swinging toward expansion." American Bar Association, *Resolution and Report 607*, August 2024, https://www.americanbar.org/content/dam/aba/directories/policy/annual-2024/607-annual-2024.pdf.
32 "It has been variously estimated . . ." Matthew Miller, Yifan Zhang, David M. Studdert, and Sonja Swanson, "Updated Estimate of the Number of Extreme Risk Protection Orders Needed to Prevent 1 Suicide," *JAMA Network Open* 7, no. 6 (2024): 1, e2414864, https://doi.org/10.1001/jamanetworkopen.2024.14864.
32 "the federal categorical restriction . . ." Fredrick E. Vars, Benjamin Meadows, and Griffin Edwards, "Slipping Through the Cracks? The Impact of Reporting Mental Health Records to the National Firearm Background Check System," *Journal of Economic Behavior and Organization* 195 (March 2022): 62–63, https://doi.org/10.1016/j.jebo.2021.12.002.
32 "A 2024 systematic review . . ." "The Effects of Extreme-Risk Protection Orders," RAND, updated July 16, 2024, https://www.rand.org/research/gun-policy/analysis/extreme-risk-protection-orders.html.

33 "the first peer respite . . ." Legislative Analysis and Public Policy Association, *Peer Respites as an Alternative to Hospitalization* (February 2021), 1, https://legislative analysis.org/wp-content/uploads/2021/02/Peer-Respites-as-an-Alternative-to-Hospitilzation-FINAL.pdf.

33 "nearly three million . . ." U.S. Census Bureau, "Census Reporter Profile Page for Charlotte–Concord–Gastonia, NC–SC Metro Area," Census Reporter, 2023, https://censusreporter.org/profiles/31000US16740-charlotte-concord-gastonia-nc-sc-metro-area/.

CHAPTER 3

34 "There are now . . . prison in the United States." Treatment Advocacy Center: Office of Research and Public Affairs, *Serious Mental Illness (SMI) Prevalence in Jails and Prisons*, 2016, 1, https://www.tac.org/wp-content/uploads/2023/11/smi-in-jails-and-prisons.pdf.

34 "The rate of mental illness . . ." Laura M. Maruschak, Jennifer Bronson, and Mariel Alper, *Indicators of Mental Health Problems Reported by Prisoners* (U.S. Department of Justice, 2021), 1, https://bjs.ojp.gov/sites/g/files/xyckuh236/files/media/document/imhprpspi16st.pdf; "Mental Illness," National Institute of Mental Health, accessed June 6, 2025, https://www.nimh.nih.gov/health/statistics/mental-illness.

34 "One 2015 study . . ." Jeffrey W. Swanson, E. Elizabeth McGinty, Seena Fazel, and Vickie M. Mays, "Mental Illness and Reduction of Gun Violence and Suicide: Bringing Epidemiological Research to Policy," *Annals of Epidemiology* 25, no. 5 (2015): 372, https://doi.org/10.1016/j.annepidem.2014.03.004.

34 "after controlling for these . . ." Henry J. Steadman, Edward P. Mulvey, John Monahan, Pamela Clark Robbins, Paul S. Appelbaum, Thomas Grisso, Loren Roth, and Erik Silver, "Violence by People Discharged from Acute Psychiatric Inpatient Facilities and by Others in the Same Neighborhoods," *Archives of General Psychiatry* 55, no. 5 (1998): 393, doi:10.1001/archpsyc.55.5.393.

35 "About half . . ." Paula M. Ditton, "Mental Health and Treatment of Inmates and Probationers," *Bureau of Justice Statistics Special Report*, July 1999.

35 "In April 2019 . . . what she really needed was help." Robbins v. State, No. C-07-CR-19-000726, 2023 WL 2965785 (App. Ct. Md. Apr. 17, 2023).

36 "Overall, about a quarter . . ." Wendy Sawyer and Peter Wagner, "Mass Incarceration: The Whole Pie 2025," Prison Policy Initiative, March 11, 2025, https://www.prisonpolicy.org/reports/pie2025.html.

36 "A 2012 report . . ." Council of State Governments Justice Center, *Improving Outcomes for People with Mental Illnesses Involves with New York City's Criminal Court and Correction Systems* (2012), 3, https://csgjusticecenter.org/wp-content/uploads/2020/02/CTBNYC-Court-Jail_7-cc.pdf.

37 "A small minority of jails . . ." "Mental Health Treatment While Incarcerated," National Alliance on Mental Illness, accessed June 6, 2025, https://www.nami.org/advocacy/policy-priorities/improving-health/mental-health-treatment-while-incarcerated/#:~:text=.

37 "Often, jails administer . . ." Laura Hawks and Emily Wang, "Medication Access in Prisons and Jails—Some Answers, More Questions," *JAMA Health Forum* 4, no. 4 (2023): 1, https://doi.org/10.1001/jamahealthforum.2023.0167.

37 "One recent report . . ." Solitary Watch and Unlock the Box Campaign, *Calculating Torture: Analysis of Federal, State, and Local Data Showing More Than 122,000 People in Solitary Confinement in U.S. Prisons and Jails* (Solitary Watch, 2023), 4, https://solitarywatch.org/wp-content/uploads/2023/05/Calculating-Torture-Report-May-2023-R2.pdf.

37 "Another recent study . . ." Jessica T. Simes, Bruce Western, and Angela Lee, "Mental Health Disparities in Solitary Confinement," *Criminology* 60, no. 3 (2022): 538, https://doi.org/10.1111/1745-9125.12315.

37 "It is not surprising . . ." Fatos Kaba, Andrea Lewis, Sarah Glowa-Kollisch, James Hadler, David Lee, Howard Alper, Daniel Selling, Ross MacDonald, Angela Solimo, Amanda Parsons, and Homer Venters, "Solitary Confinement and Risk of Self-Harm Among Jail Inmates," *American Journal of Public Health* 104, no. 3 (2014): 442, https://doi.org/10.2105/AJPH.2013.301742.

37 "The suicide rate . . . more deadly." David E. Patton and Fredrick E. Vars, "Jail Suicide by Design," *UCLA Law Review* 68 (2020): 83, https://www.uclalawreview.org/wp-content/uploads/securepdfs/2020/05/Vol-68-Patton-Vars.pdf.

38 "Joshua Marsh. . . . long since been released." Esmy Jimenez, "Wait Times for Mental Health Services in WA Jails Worsen as Fines Spiral," *Seattle Times*, November 6, 2022, https://www.seattletimes.com/seattle-news/mental-health/wait-times-for-mental-health-services-in-wa-jails-worsen-as-fines-spiral/.

39 "By 2017 . . ." Doris A. Fuller, Elizabeth Sinclair, H. Richard Lamb, James D. Cayce, and John Snook, *Emptying the "New Asylums": A Beds Capacity Model to Reduce Mental Illness Behind Bars* (Treatment Advocacy Center Office of Research and Public Affairs, 2017), 24–25, https://www.tac.org/reports_publications/emptying-the-new-asylums-a-beds-capacity-model-to-reduce-mental-illness-behind-bars/.

39 "Alabama . . . 155 days in another." Hunter v. Boswell, No. 2:16cv798-MHT, 2021 WL 1095977, at *1 (M.D. Ala. Mar. 22, 2021).

39 "The endless delays . . ." Lindsey Devers, *Plea and Charge Bargaining: Research Summary* (U.S. Department of Justice Bureau of Justice Assistance, 2011), 1, https://bja.ojp.gov/sites/g/files/xyckuh186/files/media/document/pleabargainingresearchsummary.pdf.

39 "In 1962 . . . the principle applies to mental illness." Robinson v. California, 370 U.S. 660, 666, 668 (1962).

40 "*Clark v. Arizona* is a good example . . . mens rea and Clark's conviction." Clark v. Arizona, 548 U.S. 735, 743–45 (2006).

41 "In *Kahler v. Kansas* . . ." Kahler v. Kansas, 589 US 271, 274 (2020).

42 "At oral argument . . . answer to Breyer's question." Transcript of Oral Argument at 38–40, *Kahler*, 589 U.S. 271 (No. 18-6135).

43 "Fewer than 1 percent . . ." Lisa Callahan, Henry J. Steadman, Margaret A. Mc-Greevy, and Pamela Clark Robbins, "The Volume and Characteristics of Insanity

Defense Pleas: An Eight-State Study," *Bulletin of the American Academy of Psychiatry and the Law* 19, no. 4 (1991): 331, https://www.researchgate.net/publication/21370218_The_Volume_and_Characteristics_of_Insanity_Defense_Pleas_An_Eight-State_Study.

43 "In the case *Durham v. United States* . . . 'unsound mind.'" Durham v. United States, 214 F.2d 862, 864 (D.C. Cir. 1954).

43 "For his insanity defense . . . either option (a) or (b)." *Durham*, 214 F.2d at 865–66.

44 "Specifically, Bazelon redefined . . ." *Durham*, 214 F.2d at 874–75.

44 "Eighteen years later . . ." United States v. Brawner, 471 F.2d 969, 1006 (D.C. Cir. 1972), *superseded by statute*, Insanity Defense Reform Act of 1984, 18 U.S.C. §§ 17, 4241-47, *as recognized in* Shannon v. United States, 512 U.S. 573 (1994).

44 "A disappointed Judge Bazelon . . . would do any better." *Brawner*, 471 F.2d at 1010, 1013 (Bazelon, C. J., concurring in part).

44 "Under the replacement standard . . ." *Brawner*, 471 F.2d at 992 (majority opinion).

44 "Research has shown . . ." George L. Blau and Richard A. Pasewark, "Statutory Changes and the Insanity Defense: Seeking the Perfect Insane Person," *Law & Psychology Review* 18 (1994): 85.

44 "Unlike with a prison term . . ." Mac McClelland, "When 'Not Guilty' Is a Life Sentence," *New York Times*, September 27, 2017, https://www.nytimes.com/2017/09/27/magazine/when-not-guilty-is-a-life-sentence.html.

45 "Defendants who raise . . ." Michael L. Perlin, "Myths, Realities, and the Political World: The Anthropology of Insanity Defense Attitudes," *Bulletin of the American Academy of Psychiatry and the Law* 24, no. 1 (1996): 12, https://digitalcommons.nyls.edu/cgi/viewcontent.cgi?article=2233&context=fac_articles_chapters.

45 "Jamie Lee Wallace . . ." Amy Yurkanin, "SPLC: Emergency Action Needed After Suicide of Mentally Ill Alabama Prison Inmate," AL.com, December 22, 2016, https://www.al.com/news/2016/12/attorneys_seek_emergency_actio.html; Jeremy Gray, "The Sad, Short, Violent Life of Jamie Lee Wallace: We Fail Those Who Most Need Help," AL.com, December 23, 2016, https://www.al.com/opinion/2016/12/the_sad_short_violent_life_of.html.

45 "In 2014, Wallace agreed . . ." Class Action Complaint for Declaratory and Injunctive Relief, Braggs v. Dunn, 257 F. Supp. 3d 1171 (2017) (No. 2:14-CV-00601), 2014 WL 2884835.

46 "Wallace's testimony and death . . ." Liability Opinion and Order as to Phase 2A Eighth Amendment Claim at 299, *Braggs*, 257 F. Supp. 3d 1171 (No. 2:14-CV-00601).

47 "The one person . . ." Beth Shelburne, "What Happened to Jamie Lee Wallace?," WBRC News, July 5, 2017, https://www.wbrc.com/story/35819522/what-happened-to-jamie-lee-wallace/.

47 "In 1994, a federal judge . . ." Coleman v. Wilson, 912 F. Supp. 1282, 1297 (E.D. Cal. 1995).

47 "California failed to correct . . . not covered by the court order." Brown v. Plata, 563 U.S. 493, 500, 538 (2011).

47 "Take, for example . . . in the community or in hospital." Hillary Kunis, *Mental Health San Francisco Implementation Plan* (San Francisco Department of Public Health, 2023), 13, https://www.sf.gov/sites/default/files/2023-02/DPH%20MHSF%20Implementation%20Report%202023_0.pdf.

48 "An independent crisis center . . . out of emergency departments." Margaret Kates, "Crisis Centers and Clinics: New Mental Health Care Models Attempt to Fill Gaps in Alabama System," AL.com, October 5, 2022, https://www.al.com/news/2022/10/crisis-centers-and-clinics-new-mental-health-care-models-attempt-to-fill-gaps-in-alabama-system.html.

49 "Jurisdictions that have moved away . . ." Thomas Hanna, "The Facts on New Jersey Bail Reform," Arnold Ventures, March 1, 2023, https://www.arnoldventures.org/stories/the-facts-on-new-jersey-bail-reform.

49 "On the other hand . . ." Leah G. Pope, Tehya Boswell, Adria Zern, Blake Erickson, and Michael T. Compton, "Failure to Appear: Mental Health Professionals' Role Amidst Pretrial Justice Reform," *Psychiatric Services* 73, no. 7 (2022): 810, https://doi.org/10.1176/appi.ps.202100252.

49 "The reasons . . . lower costs than incarceration." Evelyn F. McCoy, Azhar Gulaid, Nkechi Erondu, and Janeen Buck Willison, *Removing Barriers to Pretrial Appearance* (Urban Institute, 2021), 2, https://www.urban.org/sites/default/files/publication/104177/removing-barriers-to-pretrial-appearance_0.pdf.

50 "One way or another . . . recovery, not punishment." Derek Denckla and Greg Berman, *Rethinking the Revolving Door: A Look at Mental Illness in the Courts* (Center for Court Innovation, 2001), 2, https://www.innovatingjustice.org/wp-content/uploads/2001/07/rethinkingtherevolvingdoor.pdf.

51 "Amy Geisel was one of the first . . . creating new programs" "Amy Graduates from Therapeutic Mental Health Court and Soars to Help Others," Pioneer Human Services, accessed June 7, 2025, https://pioneerhumanservices.org/success-stories/amy-graduates-theraputic-mental-health-court-and-soars-to-help-others/.

51 "In 2012 . . . Pennsylvania correctional institutions." Lynn Patrone, "Peer Support Behind Bars in Pennsylvania," *GAINS Center Newsletter*, August 2017, https://t.e2ma.net/pages/1776550/2958.

52 "As of August 2024 . . ." Elizabeth Hinton, Akash Pillai, and Amaya Diana, "Section 1115 Waiver Watch: Medicaid Pre-Release Services for People Who Are Incarcerated," KFF, August 19, 2024, https://www.kff.org/medicaid/issue-brief/section-1115-waiver-watch-medicaid-pre-release-services-for-people-who-are-incarcerated/.

52 "In contrast, treatment . . ." Sarah Youn, Belinda L. Guadagno, Linda K. Byrne, Amity E. Watson, Sean Murrihy, and Sue M. Cotton, "Systematic Review and Meta-Analysis: Rates of Violence During First-Episode Psychosis (FEP)," *Schizophrenia Bulletin* 50, no. 4 (2024):766, https://doi.org/10.1093/schbul/sbae010.

52 "As one researcher states . . ." Youn et al., "Systematic Review and Meta-Analysis," 766–67.

CHAPTER 4

54 "In 1963 . . . mental healthcare has never recovered." Mark Moran, "Vision Revisited: 50 Years of the Community Health Care Act," *Psychiatry Online* 48, no. 22 (2013): 1, https://doi.org/10.1176/appi.pn.2013.11b24.

54 "For example, Diane Wilson . . ." Wilson v. Formigoni, 42 F.3d 1060 (7th Cir. 1994).

55 "First, 'voluntary' admissions . . ." Ted Lutterman, Robert Shaw, William Fisher, and Ronald Manderscheid, *Trend in Psychiatric Inpatient Capacity, United States and Each State, 1970 to 2014* (National Association of State Mental Health Program Directors, 2017), 17, https://www.nri-inc.org/media/1319/tac-paper-10-psychiatric-inpatient-capacity-final-09-05-2017.pdf.

55 "In recent years . . . main reasons they give." "Reducing the Economic Burden of Unmet Mental Health Needs," WH.gov, May 31, 2022, https://bidenwhitehouse.archives.gov/cea/written-materials/2022/05/31/reducing-the-economic-burden-of-unmet-mental-health-needs/.

55 "Most psychiatrists . . ." Tara F. Bishop, Matthew J. Press, Salomeh Keyhani, and Harold Alan Pincus, "Acceptance of Insurance by Psychiatrists and the Implications for Access to Mental Health Care," *JAMA Psychiatry* 71, no. 2 (2014): 176, https://jamanetwork.com/journals/jamapsychiatry/fullarticle/1785174.

56 "Medicaid accounts for . . ." Roberta Baker, "How NH's Mental Health Care System Closed Gaps But Why a 'Tremendous Amount' Remain," Seacoastonline, March 26, 2023, https://www.seacoastonline.com/in-depth/news/2023/03/26/new-hampshire-mental-health-care-gaps-staffing-shortfalls-education-opportunity-increase-services/70038626007/.

56 "One example of a high-intensity . . . into their communities." Gary R. Bond and Robert E. Drake, "The Critical Ingredients of Assertive Community Treatment," *World Psychiatry* 14, no. 2 (2015): 240, https://doi.org/10.1002/wps.20234.

57 "There is overwhelming evidence . . ." Marina Dietrich, Claire B. Irving, Hanna Bergman, Mariam A. Khokhar, Bert Park, and Max Marshall, "Intensive Case Management for Severe Mental Illness (Review)," *Cochrane Database of Systematic Reviews* 1 (2017): 34–35, CD007906, https://doi.org/10.1002/14651858.CD007906.pub3.

57 "Studies find positive outcomes . . . and client satisfaction." Dietrich et al., "Intensive Case Management," 35–40.

57 "Research finds that ACT teams . . . therapeutic relationships." Jennifer L. Wright-Berryman, Alan B. McGuire, and Michelle P. Salyers, "A Review of Consumer-Provided Services on Assertive Community Treatment and Intensive Case Management Teams: Implications for Future Research and Practice." *Journal of the American Psychiatric Nurses Association* 17, no. 1 (2011): 41, https://doi.org/10.1177/1078390310393283.

57 "A 2015 randomized study . . ." Matthew Chinman, Rebecca S. Oberman, Barbara H. Hanusa, Amy N. Cohen, Michelle P. Salyers, Elizabeth W. Twamley, and Alexander S. Young, "A Cluster Randomized Trial of Adding Peer Specialists to Intensive Case Management Teams in the Veterans Health Administration," *Journal of Behavioral Health Services & Research* 42, no. 1 (2015): 113, https://doi.org/10.1007/s11414-013-9343-1.

58 "Studies have found . . ." Eric P. Slade, John F. McCarthy, Marcia Valenstein, Stephanie Visnic, and Lisa B. Dixon, "Cost Savings from Assertive Community Treatment Services in an Era of Declining Psychiatric Inpatient Use," *Health Services Research* 48, no. 1 (2013): 210, https://doi.org/10.1111/j.1475-6773.2012.01420.x.

59 "A 2023 randomized study . . ." Daniel Maeng, Zhi-Yang Tsun, Eric Lesch, David B. Jacobwitz, Robert L. Strawderman, Donald K. Harrington, Yue Li, Robert L. Weisman, and Steven Lamberti, "Affordability of Forensic Assertive Community Treatment Programs: A Return-on-Investment Analysis," *Psychiatric Services* 74, no. 4 (2023): 358, https://doi.org/10.1176/appi.ps.20220186.

59 "A large Canadian study . . . 'strongly agree.'" Sean A. Kidd, Lindsey George, Maria O'Connell, John Sylvestre, Helen Kirkpatrick, Gina Browne, and Lehana Thabane, "Fidelity and Recovery-Orientation in Assertive Community Treatment," *Community Mental Health Journal* 46, no. 4 (2010): 346, https://doi.org/10.1007/s10597-009-9275-7.

59 "In January 1999 . . ." Ali Watkins, "A Horrific Crime on the Subway Led to Kendra's Law. Years Later, Has It Helped?," *New York Times*, September 11, 2018, https://www.nytimes.com/2018/09/11/nyregion/kendras-law-andrew-goldstein-subway-murder.html.

59 "Under the law . . ." New York Mental Hygiene Law § 9.60 (McKinney 2025).

60 "In 1978 . . . decision is wise or unwise.'" *In re* Quackenbush, 383 A.2d 785, 789 (Morris County Ct. Prob. Div. 1978); Lane v. Candura, 376 N.E.2d 1232, 1236 (Mass. App. Ct. 1978).

61 "Two of these . . ." Tom Burns, Jorun Rugkåsa, Andrew Molodynski, John Dawson, Ksenija Yeeles, Maria Vazquez-Montes, Merryn Voysey, Julia Sinclair, and Stefan Priebe, "Community Treatment Orders for Patients with Psychosis (OCTET): A Randomized Control Trial," *Lancet* 381, no. 9878 (2013): 1627, https://doi.org/10.1016/S0140-6736(13)60107-5; Henry J. Steadman, Kostas Gounis, Deborah Dennis, Kim Hopper, Brenda Roche, Marvin Swartz, and Pamela Clark Robbins, "Assessing the New York City Involuntary Outpatient Commitment Pilot Program," *Psychiatric Services* 52, no. 3 (2001): 330, https://doi.org/10.1176/appi.ps.52.3.330.

61 "The third reported . . ." Marvin S. Swartz, Jeffrey W. Swanson, Ryan Wagner, Barbara J. Burns, Virginia A. Hiday, and Randy Borum, "Can Involuntary Outpatient Commitment Reduce Hospital Recidivism? Findings from a Randomized Trial with Severely Mentally Ill Individuals," *American Journal of Psychiatry* 156, no. 12 (1999): 1968, 1974, https://doi.org/10.1176/ajp.156.12.1968.

61 "One of the most thorough . . . the benefits from extra services." Marvin S. Swartz, Christine M. Wilder, Jeffrey W. Swanson, Richard A. Van Dorn, Pamela Clark Robbins, Henry J. Steadman, Lorna L. Moser, Allison R. Gilbert, and John Monahan, "Assessing Outcomes for Consumers in New York's Assisted Outpatient Treatment Program," *Psychiatric Services* 61, no. 10 (2010): 976, 980, https://doi.org/10.1176/ps.2010.61.10.976.

62 "Before a mandatory treatment . . ." New York Mental Hygiene Law § 9.60.

Notes

62 "In 2001, one judge . . ." *In re* Weinstock, 723 N.Y.S.2d 617, 620 (Sup. Ct. 2001).
62 "In one case . . ." *In re* William C., 880 N.Y.S.2d 317, 320-21 (App. Div. 2009).
63 "Even as New York . . . self-directed treatment goals." Ruthanne Becker, "The Mental Health Association of Westchester's Intensive and Sustained Engagement Team (INSET)," *Behavioral Health News*, July 19, 2023, https://behavioralhealthnews.org/the-mental-health-association-of-westchesters-intensive-and-sustained-engagement-team-inset/.
63 "the state legislature recently . . ." "Governor Hochul Signs Legislation to Improve Mental Health Care and Strengthen Treatment for Serious Mental Illness as Part of FY 2026 Budget," Governor Kathy Hochul, May 9, 2025, https://www.governor.ny.gov/news/governor-hochul-signs-legislation-improve-mental-health-care-and-strengthen-treatment-serious.
65 "Another approach . . ." Texas Health & Safety Code Ann. § 574.0345 (West 2025).

CHAPTER 5

69 "In the 1940s . . . 'We Are Not Alone.'" "Our Founding Story," Fountain House, accessed June 10, 2025, https://www.fountainhouse.org/about/our-history.
70 "total institutions . . ." Erving Goffman, *Asylums: Essays on the Social Situation of Mental Patients and Other Inmates* (Taylor & Francis, 2017).
70 "Research . . . increased wages." M. Usman and Joshua Seidman, *Beyond Treatment: How Clubhouses for People Living with Serious Mental Illness Transform Lives and Save Money* (Fountain House, 2024), 15, https://www.fountainhouse.org/assets/featurePost/FH_BeyondTreatment_Feb7v2.pdf.
70 "New York state is taking note . . ." "Governor Hochul Signs Legislation to Improve Mental Health Care and Strengthen Treatment for Serious Mental Illness as Part of FY 2026 Budget," Governor Kathy Hochul, May 9, 2025, https://www.governor.ny.gov/news/governor-hochul-signs-legislation-improve-mental-health-care-and-strengthen-treatment-serious.
70 "In May 2023 . . ." Julianne Holt-Lunstad and Susan Golant, eds., *Our Epidemic of Loneliness and Isolation: The U.S. Surgeon General's Advisory on the Healing Effects of Social Connection and Community* (U.S. Department of Health and Human Services, 2023), https://www.hhs.gov/sites/default/files/surgeon-general-social-connection-advisory.pdf.
70 "This is particularly true . . ." Eris F. Perese and Marilee Wolf, "Combating Loneliness Among Persons with Severe Mental Illness: Social Network Interventions' Characteristics, Effectiveness, and Applicability," *Issues in Mental Health Nursing* 26, no. 6 (2005): 591, https://doi.org/10.1080/01612840590959425.
71 "Research confirms that the clubhouse . . ." Joshua Seidman and Kevin Rice, *Brief Summary of Evidence Supporting Clubhouses* (Fountain House, 2022), 3, https://www.fountainhouse.org/assets/Brief-Summary-of-Evidence-for-Clubhouses_2022.pdf.
71 "It is therefore not surprising . . ." Holt-Lunstad and Golant, *Our Epidemic*, 71.

CHAPTER 6

79 "Over 770,000 people . . ." "HUD Releases January 2024 Point-in-Time Count Report," U.S. Department of Housing and Urban Development Archives, December 27, 2024, https://archives.hud.gov/news/2024/pr24-327.cfm.

79 "Among unhoused people . . ." Deborah K. Padgett, "Homelessness, Housing Instability and Mental Health: Making the Connections," *BJPsych Bulletin* 44, no. 5 (2020): 197, https://doi.org/10.1192/bjb.2020.49.

79 "By comparison, only . . ." "Mental Illness," National Institute of Mental Health, updated September 2024, https://www.nimh.nih.gov/health/statistics/mental-illness.

79 "Nova Honey . . . delivered to her door." Nicole Hayden, "63% of Homeless Portlanders Report Suffering from Mental Health Issues and Say They Need More Help: False Promises Survey," OregonLive, June 12, 2022, https://www.oregonlive.com/portland/2022/06/63-of-homeless-portlanders-report-suffering-from-mental-health-issues-and-say-they-need-more-help-false-promises-survey.html.

84 "These events . . . first in the 1980s," David A. Mackey, "Bernhard Goetz," *Encyclopedia Britannica*, November 3, 2024, https://www.britannica.com/biography/Bernhard-Goetz.

84 "then again in the 2020s." Kiara Alfonseca and Jason Potere, "Who Is Jordan Neely, the Man Killed in NYC Subway Chokehold Death?," ABC News, October 21, 2024, https://abcnews.go.com/US/jordan-neely-man-killed-nyc-subway-chokehold-death/story?id=114848209.

84 "In response . . . 'necessary medical care.'" Cal. Welf. & Inst. Code § 5008(h)(1)(A) (West, Westlaw through Ch. 3 of 2025 Reg. Sess.).

85 "More than a third . . ." Laurence Roy, Anne G. Crocker, Tonia L. Nicholls, Eric A. Latimer, and Andrea Reyes Ayllon, "Criminal Behavior and Victimization Among Homeless Individuals with Severe Mental Illness: A Systematic Review," *Psychiatric Services* 65, no. 6 (2014): 746, https://doi.org/10.1176/appi.ps.201200515.

85 "An interesting feature . . . newly eligible people." Trân Nguyễn, "New California Law Aims to Force People with Mental Illness or Addiction to Get Help," PBS, October 10, 2023, https://www.pbs.org/newshour/politics/new-california-law-aims-to-force-people-with-mental-illness-or-addiction-to-get-help

85 "Even within that fraction . . . suicidal thinking." Padgett, "Homelessness, Housing Instability and Mental Health," 197.

85 "The top three causes . . ." National Law Center on Homeless and Poverty, *Homelessness in America: Overview of Data and Causes* (2015), 3, https://homelesslaw.org/wp-content/uploads/2018/10/Homeless_Stats_Fact_Sheet.pdf.

85 "In 2023, California . . ." Margot Kushel and Tiana Moore, *Toward a New Understanding: The California Statewide Study of People Experiencing Homelessness* (UCSF Benioff Homelessness and Housing Initiative, 2023), 19, https://homelessness.ucsf.edu/sites/default/files/2023-06/CASPEH_Report_62023.pdf.

85 "Black people are more likely . . ." "What Is Homelessness in America?," National Alliance to End Homelessness, accessed June 16, 2025, https://endhomelessness.org/overview/.

85 "Between 22 percent and 57 percent . . ." Administration for Children and Families Office of Family Violence Prevention and Services, *Domestic Violence and Homelessness: Statistics* (2016), 2, https://acf.gov/ofvps/fact-sheet/domestic-violence-and-homelessness-statistics-2016.

85 "surveys find that . . ." National Alliance to End Homelessness, *Summary of Public Opinion Polling on Homelessness, June 2024,* 2024, 3, https://endhomelessness.org/wp-content/uploads/2024/09/Summary-of-Public-Opinion-Polling-on-Homelessness-June-2024.pdf.

85 "People systematically overestimate . . ." Amos Tversky and Daniel Kahneman, "Availability: A Heuristic for Judging Frequency and Probability," *Cognitive Psychology* 5, no. 2 (1973): 223, https://doi.org/10.1016/0010-0285(73)90033-9.

86 "'The problem of homelessness . . . still have this problem.'" April Dembosky, Amelia Templeton, and Carrie Feibel, "When Homelessness and Mental Illness Overlap, Is Forced Treatment Compassionate?," NPR, March 31, 2023, https://www.npr.org/sections/health-shots/2023/03/31/1164281917/when-homelessness-and-mental-illness-overlap-is-compulsory-treatment-compassiona.

86 "A large-scale 2023 survey . . ." Margot Kushel and Tiana Moore, *Toward a New Understanding*, 6.

86 "As I was writing . . ." City of Grants Pass v. Johnson, 603 U.S. 520, 560-61 (2024).

88 "The Housing First Model . . . keep them housed." "Homelessness Research Resources Repository: Housing First," Joint Office of Homeless Services, accessed June 16, 2025, https://omeka.pdx.edu/housingfirst.

89 "More than twenty years . . . better housing outcomes." Andrew J. Baxter, Emily J. Tweed, Srinivasa Vittal Katikireddi, and Hilary Thomson, "Effects of Housing First Approaches on Health and Well-Being of Adults Who Are Homeless or at Risk of Homelessness: Systematic Review and Meta-Analysis of Randomized Controlled Trials," *Journal of Epidemiology and Community Health* 73, no. 5 (2019): 379, https://doi.org/10.1136/jech-2018-210981.

89 "They find housing more quickly . . ." Sam Tsemberis, Leyla Gulcur, and Maria Nakae, "Housing First, Consumer Choice, and Harm Reduction for Homeless Individuals with a Dual Diagnosis," *American Journal of Public Health* 94, no. 4 (2004): 651, https://doi.org/10.2105/AJPH.94.4.651.

89 "and they report higher satisfaction . . ." Debra J. Rog, Tina Marshall, Richard H. Dougherty, Preethy George, Allen S. Daniels, Sushmita Shoma Ghose, and Miriam E. Delphin-Rittmon, "Permanent Supportive Housing: Assessing the Evidence," *Psychiatric Services* 65, no. 3 (2014): 292, https://doi.org/10.1176/appi.ps.201300261.

89 "In addition, Housing First reduces . . ." Baxter et al., "Effects of Housing First Approaches on Health," 384.

89 "reduced police, judicial, and welfare . . ." Verughese Jacob, Sajal K. Chattopadhyay, Sharon Attipoe-Dorcoo, Yinan Peng, Robert A. Hahn, Ramona Finnie, Jamaicia Cobb, Alison E. Cuellar, Karen M. Emmons, Patrick L. Remington, and the Community Preventive Services Task Force, "Permanent Supportive Housing with Housing First: Findings from a Community Guide Systematic Economic Review,"

American Journal of Preventive Medicine 62, no. 3 (2022): e195, https://doi.org/10.1016/j.amepre.2021.08.009.
89 "A 2022 review . . ." Jacob et al., "Permanent Supportive Housing with Housing First," e195.
89 "The model also includes . . ." Baxter et al., "Effects of Housing First Approaches on Health," 379.
91 "Detox programs alone fail . . ." Dean R. Gerstein and Henrick J. Harwood, eds., *Treating Drug Problems, Vol. 1: A Study of the Evolution, Effectiveness, and Financing of Public and Private Drug Treatment Systems* (National Academy Press, 1990), 176.
95 "In 2023, the City of Birmingham . . ." Greg Garrison, "Birmingham Approves Plan to Offer Tiny Shelters to the Homeless," AL.com, January 10, 2023, https://www.al.com/news/2023/01/birmingham-approves-plan-to-offer-tiny-shelters-to-the-homeless.html.
95 "but that effort . . ." Jon Paepcke, "Ensley Neighborhood Leaders Pushing Back Against Homeless Project," WVTM 13, updated April 30, 2024, https://www.wvtm13.com/article/ensley-neighborhood-leaders-pushing-back-against-homeless-project-birmingham/60641008.

CHAPTER 7

101 "Consistent with Stephanie's experience . . . mental health intervention.'" Robert E. Drake and Michael A. Wallach, "Employment is a Critical Mental Health Intervention," *Epidemiology and Psychiatric Sciences* 29 (2020): 1, e178, https://doi.org/10.1017/S2045796020000906.
102 "Estimates of the . . ." Alison Luciano and Ellen Meara, "Employment Status of People with Mental Illness: National Survey Data from 2009 and 2010," *Psychiatric Services* 65, no. 10 (2014): 1201, https://doi.org/10.1176/appi.ps.201300345; Sita Diehl, Dania Douglas, and Ron Honberg, *Road to Recovery: Employment and Mental Illness* (National Alliance on Mental Illness, 2014), 4, https://www.nami.org/wp-content/uploads/2023/08/RoadtoRecovery.pdf.
102 "A 2008 study . . ." Colleen Labbe, "Mental Disorders Cost Society Billions in Unearned Income," National Institute of Mental Health, May 7, 2008, https://www.nimh.nih.gov/news/science-updates/2008/mental-disorders-cost-society-billions-in-unearned-income.
102 "studies dating back to the 1980s . . ." John S. Straus and Larry Davidson, "Mental Disorders, Work, and Choice," in *Mental Disorder, Work Disability, and the Law*, ed. Richard J. Bonnie and John Monahan (University of Chicago Press, 1996), 110.
104 "One evidence-based . . . rehabilitation models." Matthew Modini, Leona Tan, Beate Brinchmann, Min-Jung Wang, Eoin Killackey, Nicholas Glozier, Arnstein Mykletun, and Samuel B. Harvey, "Supported Employment for People with Severe Mental Illness: Systematic Review and Meta-Analysis of the International Evidence," *British Journal of Psychiatry* 209, no. 1 (2016): 14, https://doi.org/10.1192/bjp.bp.115.165092.
105 "A 2023 analysis . . . outcomes at a lower cost." Robert E. Drake and Gary R. Bond, "Individual Placement and Support: History, Current Status, and Future

Directions," *Psychiatry and Clinical Neurosciences Reports* 2, no. 3 (2023): 5, 7, e122, https://doi.org/10.1002/pcn5.122.
105 "At the formal end of the spectrum . . ." Judith A. Cook, Pamela J. Steigman, Margaret Swarbrick, Jane K. Burke-Miller, Tania B. Laing, Laurie Vite, Jessica A. Jonikas, and Isaac Brown, "Outcomes of Peer-Provided Individual Placement and Support Services in a Mental Health Peer-Run Vocational Program," *Psychiatric Services* 74, no. 5 (2023): 480, https://doi.org/10.1176/appi.ps.20220134.
106 "The federal Americans with Disabilities Act . . . and 'working.'" Americans with Disabilities Act, definition of disability, 42 U.S.C. § 12102 (2018).
110 "Over 90 percent of U.S. employers . . ." HR.com, *Background Screening: Trends and Uses in Today's Global Economy* (Professional Background Screening Association, 2020), 5, https://pubs.thepbsa.org/pub.cfm?id=459B8AB7-0CEA-625E-0911-A4A089DE5118.
110 "In most of the country . . . illness as 'unacceptable.'" Palmer v. Circuit Court of Cook County, 117 F.3d 351, 352 (7th Cir. 1997).
111 "These courts recognize that . . . business necessity.'" Gambini v. Total Renal Care, Inc., 486 F.3d 1087, 1095 (9th Cir. 2007).
111 "An example . . . shows what's at stake" U.S. Equal Employment Opportunity Commission, *Enforcement Guidance on the ADA and Psychiatric Disabilities* (EEOC-CVG-1997-2, 1997).
113 "'Authenticity has been shown . . .'" Evelien P. M. Brouwers, "Social Stigma Is an Underestimated Contributing Factor to Unemployment in People with Mental Illness or Mental Health Issues: Position Paper and Future Directions," *BMC Psychology* 8, no. 36 (2020): 4, https://doi.org/10.1186/s40359-020-00399-0.
114 "The U.S. Department of Labor . . . correct that omission." Providing Empathetic and Effective Recovery Support Act, S. 2733 (Sept. 6, 2023).

CHAPTER 8

117 "In the United States . . . $600,000 or so." "Education Pays," U.S. Bureau of Labor Statistics, April 18, 2025, https://www.bls.gov/emp/tables/unemployment-earnings-education.htm.
117 "Education helped me . . ." Laurie Knis-Matthews, Josephine Bokara, Lorena DeMeo, Nicole Lepore, and Lauren Mavus, "The Meaning of Higher Education for People Diagnosed with a Mental Illness: Four Students Share Their Experiences," *Psychiatric Rehabilitation Journal* 31, no. 2 (2007): 110, https://doi.org/10.2975/31.2.2007.107.114.
117 "a study of the clubhouse model . . ." Jennifer Sánchez, Connie Sung, Brian N. Phillips, Molly K. Tschopp, Veronica Muller, Hui-Ling Lee, and Fong Chan, "Predictors of Perceived Social Effectiveness of Individuals with Serious Mental Illness," *Psychiatric Rehabilitation Journal* 42, no. 1 (2019): 88, https://doi.org/10.1037/prj0000321.
117 "Research has also identified . . ." Mary Elizabeth Collins, Deborah Bybee, and Carol T. Mowbray, "Effectiveness of Supportive Education for Individuals with Psychiatric Disabilities: Results from an Experimental Study," *Community*

Mental Health Journal 34, no. 6 (1998): 600, 612, https://doi.org/10.1023/a:1018763018186.

118 "One 2005 study . . . overall dropout rate." Mary Elizabeth Collins and Carol T. Mowbray, "Higher Education and Psychiatric Disabilities: National Survey of Campus Disability Services," *American Journal of Orthopsychiatry* 75, no. 2 (2005): 304, https://doi.org/10.1037/0002-9432.75.2.304.

118 "Similar disparities exist . . ." Child Mind Institute, *2016 Children's Mental Health Report* (2016), 4, https://childmind.org/wp-content/uploads/2021/09/2016-Childrens-Mental-Health-Report.pdf.

118 "Young adulthood . . ." Marco Solmi, Joaquim Radua, Miriam Olivola, Enrico Croce, Livia Soardo, Gonzalo Salazar de Pablo, Jae Il Shin, James B. Kirkbride, Jae Han Kim, Jong Yeob Kim, Andrè F. Carvalho, Mary V. Seeman, Christoph U. Correl, and Paolo Fusar-Poli, "Age at Onset of Mental Disorders Worldwide: Large-Scale Meta-Analysis of 192 Epidemiological Studies," *Molecular Psychiatry* 27 (2022): 285, https://www.nature.com/articles/s41380-021-01161-7.

118 "At the same time . . ." Ipsos, *How America Completes College* (Sallie Mae, 2024), 8–9, https://www.salliemae.com/content/dam/slm/writtencontent/Research/SLM_How-America-Completes-College-Research-report.pdf.

118 "Research shows that about half . . ." Sarah Wood, "Mental Health at College: What to Know," *U.S. News & World Report*, June 3, 2025, https://www.usnews.com/news/education-news/articles/mental-health-on-college-campuses-challenges-and-solutions.

119 "A 2019 study . . . lifetime earnings of 7 percent ($40,900)." Seth A. Seabury, Sarah Axeen, Gwyn Pauley, Bryan Tysinger, Danielle Schlosser, John B. Hernandez, Hanke Heun-Johnson, Henu Zhao, and Dana P. Goldman, "Measuring the Lifetime Costs of Serious Mental Illness and the Mitigating Effects of Educational Attainment," *Health Affairs* 38, no. 4 (2019): 652, 656–57, https://doi.org/10.1377/hlthaff.2018.05246.

119 "Other research shows . . ." Lisa B. Dixon, Howard H. Goldman, Melanie E. Bennett, Yuanjia Wang, Karen A. McNamara, Sapna J. Mendon, Amy B. Goldstein, Chien-Wen J. Choi, Rufina J. Lee, Jeffrey A. Lieberman, and Susan M. Essock, "Implementing Coordinated Specialty Care for Early Psychosis: The RAISE Connection Program," *Psychiatric Services* 66, no. 7 (2015): 691, 695, https://doi.org/10.1176/appi.ps.201400281.

120 "Participants describe staff . . ." Alicia Lucksted, Susan M. Essock, Jennifer Stevenson, Sapna J. Mendon, Ilana R. Missel, Howard H. Goldman, Amy B. Goldstein, and Lisa B. Dixon, "Client Views of Engagement in the RAISE Connection Program for Early Psychosis Recovery," *Psychiatric Services* 66, no. 7 (2015): 701, https://doi.org/10.1176/appi.ps.201400475.

120 "RAISE-ETP is not . . . with mental illness." Sandra Steingard, "The Recovery After an Initial Schizophrenia Episode (RAISE) Study: Notes from the Trenches," Mad in America, November 4, 2015, https://www.madinamerica.com/2015/11/the-raise-study-notes-from-the-trenches/.

121 "In 2015 . . . never being readmitted.'" Rachel Siegel and Vivian Wang, "Student Death Raises Questions on Withdrawal Policies," *Yale Daily News*, January 29,

2015, https://yaledailynews.com/blog/2015/01/29/student-death-raises-questions-on-withdrawal-policies/.

121 "Instead of withdrawing . . ." Stephanie Addenbrooke, "After Frantic Search, Community Mourns Luchang Wang '17," *Yale Daily News*, January 28, 2015, https://yaledailynews.com/blog/2015/01/28/after-frantic-search-community-mourns-sophomores-death/.

121 "In response, Yale . . ." Julianna Smolyn, "Yale University Reforms Reinstatement Policy," *Daily Pennsylvanian*, February 23, 2016, https://www.thedp.com/article/2016/02/yale-reinstatement-policy-changes; Anemona Hartocollis and Ellen Barry, "At Yale, a Surge of Activism Forced Changes in Mental Health Policies," *New York Times*, September 6, 2023, https://www.nytimes.com/2023/09/06/health/yale-mental-health.html.

121 "The tragedy was repeated . . . Ruth Bader Ginsburg." Natalie Kainz and Zaporah Price, "'She Was Unapologetically Herself': Communities Mourn Rachael Shaw-Rosenbaum '24," *Yale Daily News*, March 24, 2021, https://yaledailynews.com/blog/2021/03/24/she-was-unapologetically-herself-communities-mourn-rachael-shaw-rosenbaum-class-of24/.

121 "Like Luchang . . . killed herself on campus." William Wan, "What if Yale Finds Out?," *Washington Post*, November 11, 2022, https://www.washingtonpost.com/dc-md-va/2022/11/11/yale-suicides-mental-health-withdrawals/.

121 "This time, Yale students . . ." Class Action Complaint for Declaratory and Injunctive Relief at 1, 4, Elis for Rachael, Inc. v. Yale Univ., No. 3:22-CV-01517 (D. Conn. Nov. 30, 2022).

122 "A 2023 settlement agreement . . . must still move out." Joint Motion for Approval of Individual Settlement and for Continuing Jurisdiction at 16–18, *Elis for Rachael, Inc.*

122 "fellow Ivy Princeton . . ." Katy S. Griem and Graham R. Weber, "Universities Acknowledge a Mental Health Crisis. Why Is Action So Complicated?," *Harvard Crimson*, April 20, 2024, https://www.thecrimson.com/article/2024/4/20/mental-health-legal-scrut/.

122 "Law professor Susan Stefan . . . powers that be.'" Griem and Weber, "Universities Acknowledge a Mental Health Crisis."

123 "Here's how Evan . . . go back home.'" Shannon M. Blajeski, Vanessa V. Klodnick, Nybelle Caruso, and Tamara G. Sale, "How Early Stigmatizing Experiences, Peer Connections, and Peer Spaces Influenced Pathways to Employment or Education After a First-Episode of Psychosis," *Psychiatric Rehabilitation Journal* 45, no. 2 (2022): 148, https://doi.org/10.1037/prj0000502.

123 "A 2022 review article . . ." Jérémie Richard, Reid Rebinsky, Rahul Suresh, Serena Kubic, Adam Carter, Jasmyn E. A. Cunningham, Amy Ker, Kayla Williams, and Mark Sorin, "Scoping Review to Evaluate the Effects of Peer Support on the Mental Health of Young Adults," *BMJ Open* 12, no. 8 (2022): 1, e061336, https://doi.org/10.1136/bmjopen-2022-061336.

123 "In one small study . . ." Miri Krisi and Revital Nagar, "The Effect of Peer Mentoring on Mentors Themselves: A Case Study of College Students," *International*

Journal of Disability, Development and Education 70, no. 5 (2023): 803, https://doi.org/10.1080/1034912X.2021.1910934.

126 "Lean On Me is a national . . . many colleges and universities." Dana Humphrey, Marjorie Malpiede, and Zoe Ragouzeos, *Peer Programs in College Student Mental Health: An Essential Approach to Student Well-Being in Need of Structure and Support* (Ruderman Family Foundation; Mary Christie Institute, 2022), 16, https://marychristieinstitute.org/wp-content/uploads/2022/11/Peer-Programs-in-College-Mental-Health.pdf.

127 "Instead of . . . further education and a living wage." Nev Jones, Liping Tong, Shannon Pagdon, Ikenna D. Ebuenyi, Martin Harrow, Rajiv P. Sharma, and Cherise Rosen, "Using Latent Class Analysis to Investigate Enduring Effects of Intersectional Social Disadvantage on Long-Term Vocational and Financial Outcomes in the 20-Year Prospective Chicago Longitudinal Study," *Psychological Medicine* 54, no. 10 (2024): 2444–56, doi:10.1017/S0033291724000588.

CHAPTER 9

131 "Inspired by Bob Whitaker's book . . ." Robert Whitaker, *Mad in America: Bad Science, Bad Medicine, and the Enduring Mistreatment of the Mentally Ill* (Perseus Publishing, 2002).

131 "The trial court acknowledged . . ." Myers v. Alaska Psychiatric Inst., 138 P.3d 238, 240 (Alaska 2006).

132 "One of those victories . . . least intrusive means." *Myers* at 250. This case has been assigned reading in my mental health law seminar since 2009. Almost immediately when I met Faith, she was excited to point out something else we have in common: during a psychotic episode, each of us threw a sock out a window because we were delusional.

134 "Do the Mentally Ill Have a Right to Bear Arms?" Fredrick E. Vars and Amanda Adcock Young, "Do the Mentally Ill Have a Right to Bear Arms?," *Wake Forest Law Review* 48 (2013): 1.

134 "writing that first article . . ." Fredrick E. Vars, "Self-Defense Against Gun Suicide," *Boston College Law Review* 56 (2015): 1465.

135 "Suicide is very often impulsive . . ." Sheree J. Gibb, Annette L. Beautrais, and David M. Fergusson, "Mortality and Further Suicidal Behaviour After an Index Suicide Attempt: A 10-Year Study," *Australian and New Zealand Journal of Psychiatry* 39, no. 1–2 (2005): 96, https://doi.org/10.1080/j.1440-1614.2005.01514.

135 "Firearms rarely offer . . ." Andrew Conner, Deboral Azrael, and Matthew Miller, "Suicide Case-Fatality Rates in the United States, 2007 to 2014: A Nationwide Population-Based Study," *Annals of Internal Medicine* 171, no. 12 (2019): 885, https://doi.org/10.7326/M19-1324.

135 "only one empirical study . . . part of the 1990s." Jens Ludwig and Philip J. Cook, "Homicide and Suicide Rates Associated with Implementation of the Brady Handgun Violence Prevention Act," *JAMA* 284, no. 5 (2000): 585, https://doi.org/10.1001/jama.284.5.585.

136 "Three economists and I . . . increase in non-gun suicide." Griffin Edwards, Erik Nesson, Josh Robinson, and Fredrick Vars, "Looking Down the Barrel of a Loaded Gun: The Effect of Mandatory Handgun Purchase Delays on Homicide and Suicide," *Economic Journal* 128, no. 616 (2018): 3133–34, https://doi.org/10.1111/ecoj.12567; Michael Luca, Deepak Malhotra, and Christopher Poliquin, "Handgun Waiting Periods Reduce Gun Deaths," *Proceedings of the National Academy of Sciences* 114, no. 46 (2017): 12162, https://doi.org/10.1073/pnas.1619896114; Keith Hawton, Duleeka Knipe, and Jane Pirkis, "Restriction of Access to Means Used for Suicide," in "A Public Health Approach to Suicide Prevention," special issue, *Lancet Public Health* 9, no. 10 (2024): e798, https://doi.org/10.1016/S2468-2667(24)00157-9.

136 "Around the same time . . . said they would sign up." Fredrick E. Vars, Cheryl B. McCullumsmith, Richard C. Shelton, and Karen L. Cropsey, "Willingness of Mentally Ill Individuals to Sign Up for a Novel Proposal to Prevent Firearm Suicide," *Suicide and Life-Threatening Behavior* 47, no. 4 (2017): 483, https://doi.org/10.1111/sltb.12302.

136 "I wrote an op-ed . . ." Fredrick Vars, "A Gun Registry That Could Prevent Suicide," *Washington Post*, January 18, 2017, https://www.washingtonpost.com/opinions/a-no-guns-list-that-could-prevent-suicide/2017/01/13/b87db192-b5c4-11e6-959c-172c82123976_story.html.

136 "The state can impose . . ." Alaska Stat. Ann. §§ 47.30.730(a)(2), .735(d), .755(b) (West 2025).

136 "Jim argued in a later case . . . 'meet its burden in this case.'" *In re* Naomi B., 435 P.3d 918, 923, 933-34 (Alaska 2019).

137 "However, if there is an 'imminent threat'. . ." *Myers*, 138 P.3d 238, 248 (Alaska 2006).

137 "Off to the room . . . I was traumatized." Faith is not unusually sensitive. One study found that half of female rape victims see a male examiner as extremely problematic. Linda E. Ledray, *Evidence Collection and Care of the Sexual Assault Survivor: The SANE-SART Response* (Violence Against Women Online Resources, 2001), 4, https://vawnet.org/material/forensic-evidence-collection-and-care-sexual-assault-survivor-sane-sart-response.

138 "First, the bill . . . became law in 2008." Mentally Ill Persons—Hospitals—Medical Care and Treatment, 2008 Alaska Sess. Laws ch. 59, § 1(a), (b)(1), (c)(1), (c)(3) (codified at Alaska Stat. Ann. § 18.20.095(a), (b)(1), (c)(1), (c)(3) (West, Westlaw through ch. 6 and ch. 8 of 2025 1st Reg. Sess. of 34th Leg.).

139 "Perhaps the highest-profile example . . . twice after his disclosure." "The Thomas Eagleton Affair Haunts Candidates Today," NPR, August 4, 2012, https://www.npr.org/2012/08/04/157670201/the-thomas-eagleton-affair-haunts-candidates-today.

139 "In 1994, candidate Lynn Rivers . . . bipolar member of Congress." Rebecca Baird-Remba, "Life After Congress: Lynn Rivers," Roll Call, December 20, 2012, https://rollcall.com/2012/12/20/life-after-congress-lynn-rivers/; Gianna Melillo and Alejandra O'Connell-Domenech, "8 Lawmakers Who Have Publicly

Struggled with Mental Health," *The Hill,* February 16, 2023, https://thehill.com/changing-america/well-being/mental-health/3862175-8-lawmakers-who-have-publicly-struggled-with-mental-health/.

139 "Congressman Seth Moulton . . ." "Representative Seth Moulton," Congress.gov, accessed June 25, 2025, https://www.congress.gov/member/seth-moulton/M001196.

139 "He has spoken publicly . . . 988 mental health hotline." "Moulton Announces Launch of 988 Suicide and Crisis Lifeline," Seth Moulton, July 14, 2022, https://moulton.house.gov/news/press-releases/moulton-announces-launch-988-suicide-and-crisis-lifeline.

139 "In April 2019 . . . crowded Democratic primary field." Samantha Sergi, "Democratic Presidential Hopeful Rep. Seth Moulton Drops Out of 2020 Race," ABC News, August 23, 2019, https://abcnews.go.com/Politics/democratic-presidential-hopeful-rep-seth-moulton-drops-2020/story?id=65110454.

139 "In 2023 . . . returned to the Senate floor." Scott Detrow and Barbara Sprunt, "John Fetterman Wants to 'Pay It Forward' by Speaking Openly About His Depression," NPR, April 20, 2023, https://www.npr.org/2023/04/20/1171052245/john-fetterman-wants-to-pay-it-forward-by-speaking-openly-about-his-depression.

143 "I have elsewhere described . . ." Ian Ayres and Fredrick E. Vars, "Laboratories of Democracy," in *Weapon of Choice: Fighting Gun Violence While Respecting Gun Rights* (Harvard University Press, 2020), 39.

144 "Her 1978 book . . ." Judi Chamberlin, *On Our Own: Patient-Controlled Alternatives to the Mental Health System* (Hawthorn Books, 1978).

144 "Diana Chao . . . letters to no one in particular." "Suicide Survivor Offers Lifeline to Youth Through 'Letters to Strangers' Volunteerism," Points of Light, April 29, 2021, https://www.pointsoflight.org/awards/suicide-survivor-offers-lifeline-to-youth-through-letters-to-strangers-volunteerism/.

144 "In 2013, Diana started . . ." Jennifer Yoshikoshi, "Diana Chao: Changing the World for Mental Health," My Hero, May 15, 2023, https://myhero.com/diana-chao-changing-the-world-for-mental-health.

144 "'Letters to Strangers' (L2S) . . . advocates for legislation." *Youth-for-Youth Mental Health Guidebook.*" "About," Letters to Strangers, accessed June 25, 2025, https://www.letterstostrangers.org/about; "Donate," Letters to Strangers, accessed June 25, 2025, https://www.letterstostrangers.org/donate.

145 "In 2019, L2S published . . ." "Youth-for-Youth Mental Health Guidebook (Digital – Color)," Letters to Strangers, accessed June 25, 2025, https://www.letterstostrangers.org/product-page/youth-for-youth-mental-health-guidebook-digital-color.

145 "Seventy years before . . . PAIMI Act." Our History, Mental Health America, accessed June 25, 2025, https://mhanational.org/our-history/.

145 "In 1986, responding to . . ." "The History of P&As," Disability Rights New Jersey, accessed June 27, 2025, https://disabilityrightsnj.org/who-we-are/the-history-of-pas/#:~:text=Congress%20created%20the%20Protection%20and

%20Advocacy%20for,services%20provided%20to%20individuals%20with%20other%20disabilities.
145 "The Act expanded . . . family members of such individuals." Protection and Advocacy for Mentally Ill Individuals Act of 1986, Pub. L. No. 99-319, § 105(a)(6)(B), 100 Stat. 478, 481 (1986).
146 "That percentage was later increased . . . 42 U.S.C. § 10805(a)(6)(C); PAIMI Rule, 42 C.F.R. § 51.23(b)(1)-(2) (2024) and the PAIMI Rules at 42 CFR 51.23(b)(2), (3) and (c).
146 "A 2011 independent evaluation . . . programs receive insufficient funding." Human Services Research Institute Evaluation Team, *Evaluation of the Protection and Advocacy for Individuals with Mental Illness (PAIMI) Program: Phase III; Evaluation Report* (U.S. Department of Health and Human Services; Substance Abuse and Mental Health Services Administration, 2011), 12, 94–95, 97, https://library.samhsa.gov/sites/default/files/pep12-evalpaimi.pdf.
146 "By 2010, over forty states . . . no budget-making authority." Thomas J. Ruter and Peggy Swarbrick, *Consumer Involvement with State Mental Health Authorities*, ed. John Allen, Alan Q. Radke, and Joe Parks (National Association of Consumer/Survivor Mental Health Administrators; National Association of State Mental Health Program Directors Medical Directors Council, 2010), 21, https://web.archive.org/web/20150907024133/https://www.nasmhpd.org/sites/default/files/Consumer%20Involvement%20with%20Persons%20with%20SMI%20Final%20Part%201...rev(2).pdf#expand.
147 "U.S. District Judge . . . terminated by any court." *Wyatt ex rel. Rawlins v. Sawyer*, 219 F.R.D. 529, 533 (M.D. Ala. 2004).
147 "Trump once publicly mocked . . ." Maggie Haberman, "Donald Trump Says His Mocking of *New York Times* Reporter Was Misread," *New York Times*, November 26, 2015, https://www.nytimes.com/2015/11/27/us/politics/donald-trump-says-his-mocking-of-new-york-times-reporter-was-misread.html.
148 "The 'PEER Support Act' would . . ." Providing Empathetic and Effective Recovery Support Act, H.R. 7212, 118th Congress § 4 (2024).
148 "Paolo left . . . productive lives in our communities." Paolo del Vecchio, "Trump's Mental Health and Addiction Problem," STAT, April 21, 2025, https://www.statnews.com/2025/04/21/samhsa-elimination-trump-kennedy-rfk-jr-substance-abuse-mental-health-aha/.
149 "in a first-of-its-kind bill . . . not one member, three." H.R. 1541, 68th Leg., 2023 Reg. Sess. (Wash. 2024) (enacted).
149 "The origin story . . . 'Nothing About Us Without Us Act.'" Drew Mikkelsen, "'Nothing About Us Without Us' Act Would Require More Representation on Legislative Task Forces, Workgroups," KREM2, February 8, 2023, https://www.krem.com/article/news/politics/nothing-about-us-without-us-act-representation-legislative-work-groups/281-39fba8fb-880c-4745-baad-7d2ee7709b7c.
152 "One advocate estimated in 2018 . . ." Matt Vasilogambros, "Thousands Lose Right to Vote Under 'Incompetence' Laws," Stateline, March 21, 2018, https://stateline.org/2018/03/21/thousands-lose-right-to-vote-under-incompetence-laws/.

152 "before a 2010 amendment . . ." Andrew Oxford, "New Mexico Supreme Court Affirms Amendment Ending Ban on 'Idiot' Voters," *Santa Fe New Mexican*, September 14, 2016, https://www.santafenewmexican.com/news/local_news/new-mexico-supreme-court-affirms-amendment-ending-ban-on-idiot-voters/article_bccc0ead-49e3-5d69-85d9-2dc48d42e064.html.
152 "The Arizona Constitution . . . starts with the right to vote." *In re* Wood, 551 P.3d 1163, 1169, 1172 (Ariz. Ct. App. 2024).
152 "Two Rutgers University professors . . ." Lisa Schur and Douglas Kruse, *Fact Sheet: Disability and Voter Turnout in the 2020 Elections* (Rutgers University; Election Assistance Commission, 2021), 3, https://www.eac.gov/sites/default/files/document_library/files/Fact_sheet_on_disability_and_voter_turnout_in_2020_0.pdf.
153 "The National Disability Rights Network offered . . . signals a missed opportunity." National Disability Rights Network, *Findings from 2020 Election Omnibus Survey* (2020), 1, https://www.ndrn.org/wp-content/uploads/2020/01/NDRN-2020-Omnibus-Survey-Summary-Memo.docx.

CHAPTER 10

156 "A slave is not a mere chattel . . ." Dred Scott v. Sandford, 60 U.S. 393 (1857); dissent by Justices McLean and Curtis, p. 60 U.S. 550, https://supreme.justia.com/cases/federal/us/60/393/.
156 "The law regards man as man." Plessy v. Ferguson, 163 U.S. 537 (1896); dissent by Justice Harlan, p. 163 U. S. 559, https://supreme.justia.com/cases/federal/us/163/537/.
156 "We are saying . . ." Martin Luther King Jr., "I've Been to the Mountaintop," delivered April 3, 1968, Memphis, Tennessee, https://www.americanrhetoric.com/speeches/mlkivebeentothemountaintop.htm.
160 "stigma is defined as . . ." Bernice A. Pescosolido, Andrew Halpern-Manners, Liying Luo, and Brea Perry, "Trends in Public Stigma of Mental Illness in the US, 1996–2018," *JAMA Network Open* 4, no. 12 (2021): 2, e2140202, https://doi.org/10.1001/jamanetworkopen.2021.40202.
160 "but not always" Stephen P. Hinshaw, *The Mark of Shame: Stigma of Mental Illness and an Agenda for Change* (Oxford University Press, 2007).
161 "In a 2018 survey . . . either schizophrenia or depression." Pescosolido et al., "Trends in Public Stigma," 5.
161 "Landlords are less likely . . ." Hinshaw, *The Mark of Shame*, 100n25.
161 "One British survey . . ." Hinshaw, *The Mark of Shame*, 106n46.
162 "Over 60 percent . . . one in four Americans." Pescosolido et al., "Trends in Public Stigma," 5.
162 "a person with schizophrenia . . . a lightning strike." Sarah Youn, Belinda L. Guadagno, Linda K. Byrne, Amity E. Watson, Sean Murrihy, and Sue M. Cotton, "Systematic Review and Meta-Analysis: Rates of Violence During First-Episode Psychosis (FEP)," *Schizophrenia Bulletin* 50, no. 4 (2024): 764, https://doi.org/10.1093/schbul/sbae010.

162 "One summary of eleven studies . . ." Matthew M. Large, Christopher J. Ryan, Swaran P. Singh, Michael B. Paton, and Olav B. Nielssen, "The Predictive Value of Risk Categorization in Schizophrenia," *Harvard Review of Psychiatry* 19, no. 1 (2011): 28, https://doi.org/10.3109/10673229.2011.549770.

162 "One study of the period . . . 18 percent during the second decade." Emma McGinty, Alene Kennedy-Hendricks, Seema Chosky, and Colleen L. Barry, "Trends in News Media Coverage of Mental Illness in the United States: 1995–2014," *Health Affairs (Millwood)* 35, no. 6 (2016): 1121, 1125, https://doi.org/10.1377/hlthaff.2016.0011.

163 "A study of movies and TV shows . . ." Stacy L. Smith, Marc Choueiti, Angel Choi, Katherine Pieper, and Christine Moutier, *Mental Health Conditions in Film & TV: Portrayals that Dehumanize and Trivialize Characters* (USC Annenberg Inclusion Initiative, 2019), 4–5, https://assets.uscannenberg.org/docs/aii-study-mental-health-media_052019.pdf.

163 "Among the general population . . . a categorical failure.'" Bernice A. Pescosolido, Bianca Manago, and John Monahan, "Evolving Public Views on the Likelihood of Violence from People with Mental Illness: Stigma and Its Consequences," *Health Affairs* 38, no. 10 (2019): 1735, 1742, https://doi.org/10.1377/hlthaff.2019.00702.

163 "The rationale . . . materially affected perceived dangerousness." Erlend P. Kvaale, William H. Gottdiener, and Nick Haslam, "Biogenetic Explanations and Stigma: A Meta-Analytic Review of Associations Among Laypeople," *Social Science & Medicine* 96 (November 2013): 95, https://doi.org/10.1016/j.socscimed.2013.07.017.

164 "Research shows that knowing a friend . . ." Michelle M. Tran, Robert A. Curland, and Yan Leykin, "Association Between Treatment Seeking and Personal Knowledge of Others with Emotional or Mental Problems," *Psychiatric Services* 71, no. 4 (2020): 393, https://doi.org/10.1176/appi.ps.201900190.

164 "research shows that celebrity disclosures . . ." Petra C. Gronholm and Graham Thornicroft, "Impact of Celebrity Disclosure on Mental Health-Related Stigma," *Epidemiology and Psychiatric Sciences* 31 (2022): 2, e63, https://doi.org/10.1017/S2045796022000488.

165 "'In Our Own Voice' . . . perceptions of people with mental illness." Patrick W. Corrigan, Jennifer D. Rafacz, Julie Hautamaki, Jessica Walton, Nicolas Rüsch, Deepa Rao, Patricia Doyle, Sarah O'Brien, John Pryor, and Glenn Reeder, "Changing Stigmatizing Perceptions and Recollections About Mental Illness: The Effects of NAMI's In Our Own Voice," *Community Mental Health Journal* 46, no. 5 (2010): 517–18, https://doi.org/10.1007/s10597-009-9287-3.

165 "Other studies confirm . . ." Eunice C. Wong, Rebecca L. Collins, Jennifer L. Carully, Elizabeth Roth, Joyce S. Marks, and Jennifer Yu, *Effects of Stigma and Discrimination Reduction Trainings Conducted Under the California Mental Health Services Authority: An Evaluation of the National Alliance on Mental Illness Adult Programs* (RAND Corporation, 2015), 1, https://www.rand.org/pubs/research_reports/RR1247-1.html.

165 "Facilitators report . . ." Ken Duckworth, *You Are Not Alone: The NAMI Guide to Navigating Mental Health* (National Alliance on Mental Illness, 2022), 173.
166 "One peer put it . . ." "NAMI In Our Own Voice: Sharing Our Stories (Saturday)," posted November 16, 2022, by NAMI Maryland, YouTube, 42:49–42:57, https://youtu.be/66cxCq7DOL8?si=Fin-XPq5iQodbXR2&t=2569.
166 "NAMI has developed . . . collaborative care." Jeritt R. Tucker, Andrew J. Seidman, Julia R. Van Liew, Lisa Streyffeler, Teri Brister, Alexis Hanson, and Sydney Smith, "Effect of Contact-Based Education on Medical Student Barriers to Treating Severe Mental Illness: A Non-Randomized, Controlled Trial," *Academic Psychiatry* 44 (2020): 567, https://doi.org/10.1007/s40596-020-01290-1.
167 "NAMI Provider . . . significant positive longitudinal impact." Tucker et al., "Effect of Contact-Based Education," 566.
167 "Specifically, up to six months . . ." Julia R. Van Liew, Chunfa Jie, Jeritt R. Tucker, and Lisa Streyffeler, "Reducing Stigma and Increasing Competence Working with Mental Illness: Adaptation of a Contact-Based Program for Osteopathic Medical Students to a Virtual, Active Learning Format," *Medical Education Online* 28 (November 2022): 1, https://doi.org/10.1080/10872981.2022.2151069.

CHAPTER 11

171 "A negative sense of self . . ." Katherine Ponte, "The Many Impacts of Self-Stigma," National Alliance on Mental Illness, February 8, 2021, https://www.nami.org/recovery/the-many-impacts-of-self-stigma/#:~:text=The%20mental%20illness%20label%20is,stigma%20to%20grow%20even%20stronger.
171 "Studies show that high self-stigma . . ." Patrick W. Corrigan and Deepa Rao, "On the Self-Stigma of Mental Illness: Stages, Disclosure, and Strategies for Change," *Canadian Journal of Psychiatry* 57, no. 8 (2013): 464–69, https://doi.org/10.1177/070674371205700804; Sara Zamorano, Clara González-Sanguino, and Manuel Muñoz, "Implications of Stigma Towards Mental Health Problems on Suicide Risk in People with Mental Health Problems: A Systematic Review," *Actas Españolas de Psiquiatría* 50, no. 5 (2022): 216–25, https://pmc.ncbi.nlm.nih.gov/articles/PMC10803875/.
171 "Self-stigma can set off . . ." Patrick W. Corrigan, Johnathon E. Larson, and Nicholas Rüsch, "Self-Stigma and the 'Why Try' Effect: Impact on Life Goals and Evidence-Based Practices," *World Psychiatry* 8, no. 2 (2009): 75–81, https://doi.org/10.1002/j.2051-5545.2009.tb00218.x.
171 "Upon diagnosis . . ." Archibald, Lisa Archibald, "Mad Activists: The Language We Use Reflects Our Desire for Change," Mad in America, September 23, 2021, https://www.madinamerica.com/2021/09/mad-activists-langauge/.
172 "some advocates . . . 'psychiatric survivor' and 'mad.'" Judi Chamberlin, "The Ex-Patients' Movement: Where We've Been and Where We're Going," *Journal of Mind and Behavior* 11, nos. 3/4 (1990): 323–36, https://www.jstor.org/stable/43854095.

172 "Are Shannon Pagdon's voices . . . something different?'" Shannon Pagdon, "Why So Serious? Rethinking Dire Words," 2023 Conference on Critical Psychiatry, July 14, 2023, https://critpsych.com/blogposts/shannon-pagdon/.
173 "Refusing treatment by itself . . . evidence of anosognosia." Dinah Miller, "The Perplexing Semantics of Anosognosia," *Psychology Today*, February 21, 2018, https://www.psychologytoday.com/us/blog/committed/201802/the-perplexing-semantics-of-anosognosia.
174 "even the most effective medications . . ." Julie Garnham, Alana Munro, Claire Slaney, Marsha MacDougall, Michael Passmore, Anne Duffy, Claire O'Donovan, Andrew Teehan, and Martin Alda, "Prophylactic Treatment Response in Bipolar Disorder: Results of a Naturalistic Observation Study," *Journal of Affective Disorders* 104, nos. 1–3 (2007): 185–90, https://doi.org/10.1016/j.jad.2007.03.003.
175 "Look to . . . last place I wanted to be" Brandi Carlile, "What Can I Say," *Brandi Carlile*, Columbia, released July 12, 2005.
175 "My mind and me . . . feel alone now" Selena Gomez, "My Mind & Me," Interscope, released as a single on November 3, 2022.
175 "Sting (lithium)" Sting, "Lithium Sunset," *Mercury Falling*, A&M Records, released March 8, 1996.
175 "Kanye West (Lexapro)." Kanye West, "FML," *The Life of Pablo*, GOOD Music, released February 14, 2016.
176 "By summer's end . . . get that back." Morgan Wade, "The Night," Morgan Wade, released as a single on May 17, 2019.
176 "I'm not crazy . . . different side of me." Matchbox Twenty, "Unwell," *More Than You Think You Are*, Atlantic, released November 19, 2002.
176 "One survey in the United Kingdom . . ." Caitlin Tilley, "Listening to Taylor Swift Can Actually Affect Your Mental Health, According to Science—For Better AND Worse," DailyMail.com, October 29, 2023, https://www.dailymail.co.uk/health/article-12681477/Taylor-Swift-affect-mental-health-according-science.html. Taylor Swift had the biggest positive effect, of course, but Taylor also has a dark side, which I've written about before. Fredrick E. Vars, "Murder and Money: The Dark Side of Taylor Swift," *Duke Law Journal Online* 72 (March 2023): 146–54, https://ssrn.com/abstract=4310092.
176 "A 2021 study examined . . . 245 lives." Thomas Niederkrotenthaler, Ulrich S. Tran, Madelyn Gould, Mark Sinyor, Steven Sumner, Markus J Strauss, Martin Voracek, Benedikt Till, Sean Murphy, Frances Gonzalez, Matthew J Spittal, and John Draper, "Association of Logic's Hip Hop Song '1-800-273-8255' with Lifeline Calls and Suicides in the United States: Interrupted Time Series Analysis," *British Medical Journal* 375 (December 2021): e067726, https://doi.org/10.1136/bmj-2021-067726.
177 "Mental health stigma is stronger . . . other racial and ethnic groups." Jennifer Greif Green, Katie A. McLaughlin, Mirko Fillbrunn, Marie Fukuda, James S. Jackson, Ronald C. Kessler, Ekaterina Sadikova, Nancy A. Sampson, Corrie Vilsaint, David R. Williams, Mario Cruz-Gonzalez, and Margarita Alegría, "Barriers to Mental Health Service Use and Predictors of Treatment Drop Out: Racial/

Ethnic Variation in a Population-Based Study," *Administrative Policy in Mental Health* 47, no. 4 (2020): 606–16, https://doi.org/10.1007/s10488-020-01021-6.

178 "Studies show that women with schizophrenia . . ." Doron Amsalem, Samantha E. Jankowski, Shannon Pagdon, Linda Valeri, Stephen Smith, Lawrence Yang, John Markowitz, Roberto Lewis-Fernandez, and Lisa Dixon, "'It Is Hard to Be a Woman with Schizophrenia': Randomized Controlled Trial of a Brief Video Intervention to Reduce Public Stigma in Young Adults," *Journal of Clinical Psychiatry* 84, no. 1 (2022): 22m14534, https://doi.org/10.4088/JCP.22m14534.

181 "Over half a million Americans . . ." Ingrid D. Goldstrom, Jean Campbell, Joseph A. Rogers, David B. Lambert, Beatrice Blacklow, Marilyn J. Henderson, and Ronald W. Manderscheid, "National Estimates for Mental Health Mutual Support Groups, Self-Help Organizations, and Consumer-Operated Services," *Administration and Policy in Mental Health and Mental Health Services Research* 33, no. 1 (2006): 92–103, https://doi.org/10.1007/s10488-005-0019-x.

181 "Fountain House started . . . validated and empowered." Laura Van Tosh, Ruth O. Ralph, and Jean Campbell, "The Rise of Consumerism: A Contribution to the Surgeon General's Report on Mental Health," *Psychiatric Rehabilitation Skills* 4, no. 3 (2000): 383–409, https://cdn.kingcounty.gov/-/media/king-county/depts/dchs/behavioral-health-recovery/midd/midd/documents/the_rise_of_consumerism.pdf?la=en&rev=ced6cb0156c240a496fb0f461a10fcfa&hash=1187B42A10EE3F591EAB73A9228E6A11.

183 "A 2019 Spanish study . . . decreasing internalized prejudice." Álvaro Moraleda, Diego Galán-Casado, and Adolfo J. Cangas, "Reducing Self-Stigma in People with Severe Mental Illness Participating in a Regular Football League: An Exploratory Study," *International Journal of Environmental Research and Public Health* 16, no. 19 (2019): 3599, https://doi.org/10.3390/ijerph16193599.

183 "Research shows that this type of thinking . . ." Emily Hielscher and Geoffrey Waghorn, "Self-Stigma and Fears of Employment Among Adults with Psychiatric Disabilities," *British Journal of Occupational Therapy* 80, no. 12 (2017): 699–706, https://doi.org/10.1177/0308022617712199.

185 "It shouldn't be surprising . . ." Shinichi Nagata, Bryan McCormick, Eugene Brusilovskiy, Greg Townley, and Mark Salzer, "Disparities in Severe Loneliness Between Adults with and without a Serious Mental Illness," *Psychiatric Rehabilitation Journal* 46, no. 4 (2023): 368–72, https://doi.org/10.1037/prj0000591.

185 "Jamison argues persuasively . . ." Kay Redfield Jamison, "Could It Be Madness—This?" In *Touched with Fire: Manic-Depressive Illness and the Artistic Temperament* (Free Press, 1993), 49–99.

185 "A 2022 article reviewing . . ." Thiara Nascimento da Cruz, Evelyn V. Camelo, Antonio Egidio Nardi, and Elie Cheniaux, "Creativity in Bipolar Disorder: A Systematic Review," *Trends in Psychiatry and Psychotherapy* 44 (December 2022): e20210196, https://doi.org/10.47626/2237-6089-2021-0196.

185 "A high percentage of people . . ." Colin A. Depp, Sheeva Dev, and Lisa T. Tyler, "Bipolar Depression and Cognitive Impairment: Shared Mechanisms and New

Notes

Treatment Avenues," *Psychiatric Clinics of North America* 39, no. 1 (2016): 95–109, https://doi.org/10.1016/j.psc.2015.09.004.

186 "research shows that schizophrenia . . ." Daniel Whiting, Gautam Gulati, John R. Geddes, and Seena Fazel, "Association of Schizophrenia Spectrum Disorders and Violence Perpetration in Adults and Adolescents From 15 Countries: A Systematic Review and Meta-Analysis," *JAMA Psychiatry* 79, no. 2 (2022): 120–32, https://doi.org/10.1001/jamapsychiatry.2021.3721.

186 "The perception of dangerousness . . ." Patricia R. Owen, "Portrayals of Schizophrenia by Entertainment Media: A Content Analysis of Contemporary Movies," *Psychiatric Services* 63, no. 7 (2012): 655–59, https://doi.org/10.1176/appi.ps.201100371; Lindsey Jo Hand, "The Portrayal of Schizophrenia in Television Drama: An Experiment Asserting How Viewer Attitudes Are Affected" (Master's thesis, University of Nevada Las Vegas, 2010), https://dx.doi.org/10.34917/1448899.

186 "The Hearing Voices Network . . . to manage symptoms.'" Clyde Corentin, Caroline Fitzgerald, and John Goodwin, "Benefits of Hearing Voices Groups & Other Self-Help Groups for Voice Hearers: A Systematic Review," *Issues in Mental Health Nursing* 44, no. 4 (2023): 228–44, https://doi.org/10.1080/01612840.2023.2189953.

187 "An older man told his doctors . . . a cost, not a benefit." Zachary Ballinger, Javier Jurado Velez, and Will Rutland, "Case Report: Lilliputian Hallucinations Display Complex Pathways" (draft manuscript on file with the authors, Heersink School of Medicine, University of Alabama at Birmingham).

188 "Autonomy in treatment . . ." Julien Dubreucq, Julien Plasse, and Nicolas Franck. "Self-Stigma in Serious Mental Illness: A Systematic Review of Frequency, Correlates, and Consequences," *Schizophrenia Bulletin* 47, no. 5 (2021): 1261–87, https://doi.org/10.1093/schbul/sbaa181.

188 "Research shows that self-advocacy . . ." Jessica A. Jonikas, Dennis D. Grey, Mary Ellen Copeland, Lisa A. Razzano, Marie M. Hamilton, Carol Bailey Floyd, Walter B. Hudson, and Judith A. Cook, "Improving Propensity for Patient Self-Advocacy Through Wellness Recovery Action Planning: Results of a Randomized Controlled Trial," *Community Mental Health Journal* 49, no. 3 (2013): 260–69, https://doi.org/10.1007/s10597-011-9475-9.

188 "One study found . . . that number was 37 percent." Sophie Favre and Hélène Richard-Lepouriel, "Self-Stigma in Bipolar Disorder: A Systematic Review and Best-Evidence Synthesis," *Journal of Affective Disorders* 335 (May 2023): 273–88, https://doi.org/10.1016/j.jad.2023.05.041.

188 "In one survey, well over 50 percent . . ." Angus H. Thompson, Heather Stuart, Roger C. Bland, Julio Arboleda-Florez, Richard Warner, and Ruth A. Dickson, "Attitudes About Schizophrenia from the Pilot Site of the WPA Worldwide Campaign Against the Stigma of Schizophrenia," *Social Psychiatry and Psychiatric Epidemiology* 37, no. 10 (2002): 475–82, https://doi.org/10.1007/s00127-002-0583-2.

CONCLUSION
193 "The similarity between . . ." Saul McLeod, "Maslow's Hierarchy of Needs," *Simply Psychology*, March 14, 2025, https://www.simplypsychology.org/maslow.html.
194 "In 2024, more than one-third . . ." HRSA Health Workforce, *State of the Behavioral Health Workforce, 2024* (Health Resources and Services Administration, 2024), 1, 5, https://bhw.hrsa.gov/sites/default/files/bureau-health-workforce/state-of-the-behavioral-health-workforce-report-2024.pdf.
194 "The PEER Support Act would also codify . . ." Providing Empathetic and Effective Recovery Support Act, H.R. 2741, 119th Cong. §§ 3, 5(a) (2025).

EPILOGUE
206 "For example, one model . . . physical restraints, and seclusion." Thomas D. Begley Jr. and Andrew H. Hook, "Psychiatric Advance Directive," in *Representing the Elderly or Disabled Client* (Thomas Reuters, 2010).

INDEX

An italic "c" following a page number indicates a chart.

Abramson, Alicia, 122
accommodations, reasonable, ADA and, 106, 118, 122
acute psychosis, 3–17; personal experience of, 6–9
ADA. *See* Americans with Disabilities Act
Adams, Eric, 84
addiction: versus crime, 39–40; Rodriguez and, 80
advance directives, psychiatric, 146, 206
advocacy, 131–54, 195–96; Bryce Hospital and, 18–19; HALI and, 74; personal experience of, 140–44; retaliation for, 137; self, 188; Smith and, 100–101; types of, 151–53
Affordable Care Act, 153
Ailey, Alvin, 164
Alabama: and ACT model, 57–58; and Bryce Hospital, vii–viii, 18–20, 24–26, 157–58; and competency evaluation times, 39; and healthcare, 76; and housing issues, 87–88, 90; and integration, 157; and peer inclusion, 146; and prison conditions, 45–47; and Wyatt standards, 20
Alaska, 131–33
Aldrin, Buzz, 164
Americans with Disabilities Act (ADA), 106, 110, 122, 195
anosognosia, 173
application for employment, and self-confidence, 183–84
Arizona, 152
Assertive Community Treatment (ACT), 56–59, 89–91
Assisted Outpatient Treatment (AOT), 59–65
authenticity, 113
autonomy, 172; emergency departments and, 22; Fountain House and, 70
Autrey, Mike, vii–viii, 66

bail reform, 49–50
Bazelon, David, 44
Beckham, David, 164
Beers, Clifford, 145
behavioral health, term, 110

benefits programs: employment and, 102–3; transitional employment and, 108
Biden, Joseph, 148, 153
Biles, Simone, 164
bipolar disorder: personal experience of, viii–ix, 6–9, 133, 197–207; positive associations of, 185–86
boarding, emergency rooms and, 20–21
Brees, Katrina, 143–44
Breyer, Stephen, 42
Brock, Jon, 18–19, 26, 72–73, 105–6, 112, 148
Brown University, 124–25
Brown v. Board of Education, 156
Bryce Hospital, vii–viii, 18–20, 24–26, 157–58

CAHOOTS, 9, 48
California, 84–85
Campaign Zero, 4
Campbell, Joyce, 50–51
Canada, 188–89
Carlile, Brandi, 175
Carpenter, Leslie, 166
Carter, Jimmy, 54
cash bail, 36, 49
celebrities, and disclosure, 163–65
Chamberlin, Judi, 144
Chao, Diana, 144–45
Cimini, Dolores, 126
City of Grants Pass v. Johnson, 86–87
civil commitment. *See* involuntary hospitalization
civil rights movement, 26, 156–57
Clark, Eric, 40
Clark v. Arizona, 40–41

clozapine, 65
clubhouses. *See* Fountain House
coaches, peer, 91
coercion: ACT model and, 59; demonization and, 163; involuntary outpatient treatment and, 65–66; suicide attempts and, 27
Colbert, Stephen, 164
college. *See* higher education
Collins, Christi, 177
Colorado, 151
Committable (podcast), 31–32
community: congregate model and, 93–95; Egan and, 92; peer support in, 69–78; of practice, 114; Smith and, 99; unhoused people and, 95
community treatment models, 53–66
competency evaluations, 38–40
congregate model, 93–95
consent decree, 13
consumer, term, 146, 171
coordinated specialty care, 119–20
cost savings, 194; ACT model and, 58–59; education and, 119; EmPATH units and, 22–23; Fountain House and, 70; Housing First model and, 89–91; peer crisis response and, 11–12; recovery model and, x
COVID pandemic, 94
criminal justice system: and employment, 110; and jail, 34–52; The Other Side Academy and, 92; term, 42
crisis, 3–17; personal experience of, 3, 6–9, 197–207

Index

Crisis Assistance Helping Out On The Streets (CAHOOTS), 9, 48
crisis response teams, 9–12, 47–48
Crow, Sheryl, 164

dangerousness: combating perception of, 163; and fear, 162; and involuntary hospitalization, 25–26; statistics on, 4; weapons and, 12
decompensation, term, 37
dehumanization, 161, 190–91
deinstitutionalization, 20, 26, 54
Delaware, 158
delusions, and dangerousness, 13–16
del Vecchio, Paolo, 147–49
demonization, 162–65, 168
depression, personal experience of, 76–77, 133
deterrence, 42–43
detox programs, 91
diagnosis(/es): Fountain House and, 69; and humanity, 155; and identity, 170–71, 173–76; and isolation, 187–88; multiple, 178–79; personal experience of, 53, 69–70; with positive connotations, 185–87; and stigma, 167
difference, and stigma, 160, 167
Disability Rights Texas, 100–101
disabled, term, 171
discharge, peer support and, 27–28
disclosure of mental illness: and accommodations, 118; advantages of, 112–13; by celebrities, 163–64; and employment, 106–7, 112–15; and humanity, 158–59; personal experience of, 140–44; and politics, 139–40; small-scale, 22–25
discrimination, 105–7; anticipated, 105; disclosure and, 112; legal aspects of, 110–12; and stigma, 161; universities and, 122
disdain, and stigma, 160–61
diversion, 50–52
DMX, 164
domestic violence, and homelessness, 85
Donna's Law, 134–36, 141–44, 149–51
Downey, Robert, Jr., 164
Dred Scott v. Sandford, 156
drop outs, 118
Durham, Monte, 43
Durham v. United States, 43–44

Eagleton, Thomas, 139
education, 116–28; disclosure and, 141; and income, 117
effectiveness: of ACT model, 57; of INSET program, 63; of involuntary outpatient treatment, 61; of waiting periods for gun purchases, 135–36
Egan, Moe, 91–93
emergency department wait times, 20–23, 199
EmPATH unit, 22–23
employment, 98–115; benefits to mental health, 101–2; education and, 117; flexibility in, 195; and healthcare, 99; The Other Side Village and, 92; pay levels and stress of, 127; personal experience

of, 98–101; and self-confidence, 183–84; termination of, 110–12
employment assistance programs, limits of, 103
Equal Employment Opportunity Commission, 111
Evers, Medgar, 157–58
expectations: employment and, 127–28; hospitals and, 72; labels and, 173; Other Side Village and, 92; peer support work and, 154
Extreme Risk Protection Orders (ERPOs), 32–33

failure confessional board, 125
families, IOOV and, 165
fear: demonization and, 162–65; statistics and, 4
Fetterman, John, 139–40
first-episode psychosis (FEP), 5, 13–14
Fiscus-Surita, Anna, 28–31, 33
Floyd, George, 180
force, use of: arrestees and, 36; demonization and, 163; involuntary outpatient treatment and, 65–66; personal experience of, 202–7; police and, 4–6
forcible medication, 131–33, 137–39, 202
Forensic Assertive Community Treatment (FACT), 58–59
Fountain House, 69–71; and education, 120–21; and employment, 101, 107–9; and self-help groups, 181
Fourteenth Amendment, 156
Fox, Christina, 103, 172, 184

Frost, Ethan, 37, 178
funding issues, 194; and crisis response teams, 10; and outpatient treatment, 54, 56, 61

Gates, Bill, 164
gender, and mental illness, 178–79
Gibson, Duncan, 57–58, 94
Gish, Rick, 90–91, 94–95
Goetz, Bernard, 84
Goldstein, Andrew, 59
Gomez, Selena, 164, 175
Gottstein, Jim, 131, 136
Greenville, 81–82, 93–96
grief, and advocacy, 142
Griesel, Amy, 51
group homes, Leppala and, 71
group therapy, Smith and, 99
guardianship, and voting, 152
gun laws, 134–36, 141–44, 149–51

Hands Across Long Island (HALI), 73–74, 113–14
Harlan, John Marshall, 156
Harrell, Jennifer, 87
Harry, prince, 164
Hearing Voices Network, 186–87
Hendrix, Jimmy, 164
hiding diagnosis, costs of, 140–41
hierarchy of needs, 193
higher education, 116–28; barriers to, 118; disclosure and, 141; effects on mental health, 118; and suicide, 121–22
high school, student peer support and, 125
Hinckley, John, Jr., 44–45

Index

holistic approaches, x, 192*c*, 192–93; recommendations for, 52
Holliday, Marie, 104
homelessness, 79–97; causes of, 85; legal issues and, 86–87; Leppala and, 71; Rodriguez and, 80–83
Honey, Nova, 79
Hood, James, 157
Hope Center, 80
hospitals/hospitalization, 18–33; ACT model and, 57–58; bed shortages in, 20, 85; goal of, 203; involuntary outpatient treatment and, 61; personal experience of, 18–19, 197–207; Ramirez and, 170; recommendations for, 31–32
hotlines, 8–9, 126, 139, 176
Housing First model, 88–91
housing issues, 79–97; and self-esteem, 184–85
humanity, 155–69

identity(/ies), 170–89; changes in, 174–76, 179; education and, 117; multiple, 155, 177–81; peer support work and, 182
ill, term, 171
incapacitation, 42–43
independent crisis centers, 48–49
independent housing, 90
Individual Placement and Support model, 104–5
In Our Own Voice (IOOV), 165–66
inpatient psychiatric care. *See* hospitals
insanity: definition of, 44; versus incompetency, 38
insanity defense, 40, 43–45; avoidance of, 44–45

insight, lack of, 172–73
Intensive and Sustained Engagement Team (INSET), 63
Intensive Outpatient Programs (IOPs), 100
intent requirement, 40–41
intersectionality, 177–81
involuntary hospitalization, 24–28; effects of, 27; Gottstein and, 132–33; homelessness and, 83–84; personal experience of, 23–24, 63–64; recommendations for, 31; and treatment, 19–20; versus voluntary, 55
involuntary outpatient treatment, 59–63
involuntary treatment: Gottstein and, 131–33; personal experience of, 18, 201–2
iPads, and rural crisis response, 11
isolation: diagnosis and, 187–88; education and, 116; Fountain House and, 70–71; housing solutions and, 93–94, 185; music and, 175–76; personal experience of, 174–75. *See also* seclusion
"I WAS MYSELF" (London), 25

Jackson, Ketanji Brown, 87
jail, 34–52; ACT model and, 58–59; avoidance of, 49–52; process and conditions in, 36–39; term, 34
Jamison, Kay Redfield, 185–86
Jayapal, Pramila, 149–50
Jefferson Blount St. Clair Mental Health Authority (JBS), 71–73, 103–4, 184
jobs. *See* employment

243

Johnson, Frank, 19–20, 105
Jones, Vivian Malone, 157
Jordan, Michael, 164

Kagan, Elena, 87, 133–34
Kahler v. Kansas, 41–42
Kansas, 41–42
Kaufman-Mthimkhulu, Stefanie Lyn, 124–25
Kendra's Law, 59–63
Kennedy, John F., 54, 157
Kennedy, Robert F., Jr., 148
King, Martin Luther, Jr., 156
Koch, Ed, 84
Kruse, Douglas, 152
Kushel, Margot, 86

labels: harm of, 170; and identity, 171–74. *See also* diagnosis(/es)
Law Project for Psychiatric Rights, 131
Lean On Me, 126
least restrictive treatment, term, 62–63
legal issues: and Assisted Outpatient Treatment, 59–63; and Donna's Law, 134–36, 141–44, 149–51; and enforcement, 195; and involuntary treatment, 131–33; and jail, 34–52; and student support, 124, 126
Leppala, Sonny, 71
Letters to Strangers (L2S), 144–45
LGBTQ people, and mental illness, 180
liberty: Fountain House and, 70; involuntary medication and, 132; Kendra's Law and, 60–61

literature on lived experience, 145
lithium, 75, 197
lived experience: and ACT model, 57–58; and disclosure, 140–41; and families, 166; and homelessness, 82, 91; and peer support work, 53
Logic, 176
London, Harry, 25
loneliness, 70
Lonesome Dove (McMurtry), 60
Louisiana, 143–44
low-population density areas, crisis response in, 11

mad, term, 172
majority rule, 110–11
Mangan, Jesse, 23–24, 31–32
marginalization, Project LETS and, 125
Marsh, Joshua, 38–39
Marshall, Ann, 183
Marshall, Brandon, 3–6
Martin, Ebony, 56
Maslow, Abraham, 193
Massachusetts, 142–43
Matchbox Twenty, 176
McDonald, Laquan, 13
McMurtry, Larry, 60
media: and fear, 59, 162–63; and homelessness, 85–86; and McDonald case, 13
Medicaid, 52, 55
medication(s): and deinstitutionalization, 26–27; and education, 118; and identity, 174; Leppala and, 71–72; Myers and, 131; Myrick and, 92; Pagdon

and, 116; persistence with, 176; personal experience of, 65, 75, 77; and positive effects, 187; Smith and, 99
Melvin, Tammy, 103–4, 184
Mendoza, Vania, 10–11, 48
mens rea, 40–41
mental capacity, and involuntary hospitalization, 25–26
mental disabilities, term, 106
Mental Health America, 101, 145
mental healthcare system: in Canada, 188–89; current status of, vii, 155; illness-oriented, 191, 191*c*; in jails, 45–47; personal experience of, 74–75; whole-person, 192*c*, 192–93. *See also* hospitals/hospitalization
mental health court, 50–52
mental illness: versus crime, 39–43; and employment abilities, 104–5, 108–9; legal protections and, 40–41; personal experience of, viii–ix, 197–207; terminology on, x–xi
mental patient, term, 171
mentoring, students and, 123–24
methodology, 53
Middle Earth hotline, 126
minority rule, 111–12
Mirny, Daniel, 126
Moulton, Seth, 139
Murthy, Vivek, 70
music: for depression, 76–77; on mental illness, 175–76
Myers, Faith, 131, 137–38
Myrick, Robbie, 91–92

Napolitano, Cyrus, 69–70, 108, 182
Napper, Leslie, 178

Nathan, Donna, 143
National Alliance on Mental Illness (NAMI), 101, 140, 165–66
National Association for Rights Protection and Advocacy, 101
National Association of State Mental Health Program Directors (NASMHPD), 168
National Disability Rights Network, 153
National Rifle Association, 150–51
needs, hierarchy of, 193
Neely, Jordan, 85
neighborhoods: and housing models, 93–95; and peer crisis response, 9; and police encounters, 13; and violence, 5
Neves, Hannah, 122
New Hampshire, 21, 56
New Jersey, 49
New Mexico, 152
New York: and homelessness, 83–84; and Housing First model, 88–91; and Kendra's Law, 59–63
Nichols, Tyre, 16
Nieves, Stephanie, 101, 107–9
NIMBY, 93–95
nonadherent, term, 173
notetaker, 118
not guilty by reason of insanity, 44–45
"nothing about us without us," 144–49, 206

obsessive-compulsive disorder (OCD), vii
Office of Consumer Affairs (OCA), 146–47

Office of Recovery, 148–49, 194
O'Grady, Kathleen, 75–76
OneRoof, 87–88
open-ended questions, 64
Opportunity House, 80
The Other Side Academy, 92
The Other Side Village, 91–93
outpatient treatment models, 53–66

Pagdon, Shannon, 116–18, 120–21, 127–28
PAIMI Act, 145–46
patient, term, 171
Paxil, 180
Pedersen, Jamie, 149
peer, term, x–xi
peer bridgers, 27–28, 72
peer respite programs, 28–31; limitations of, 30–31
peer support, vii–xi, 190–96; and AOT model, 65; in community, 69–78; and crisis response, 9–12, 47–48; disclosure and, 140; and education, 121–26; effects of, 57; and emergency programs, 23; and employment, 105–6; and housing issues, 79–97; importance of, 113, 196, 205–7; and jail, 51–52; and legal system, 47–52; and mental health courts, 50–51; Pagdon and, 121; Ramirez and, 170; and self-stigma, 181–85
PEER Support Act, 114–15, 148, 194
peer support specialist, 71–73, 194
Pennsylvania, 51
Penny, Daniel, 84
personhood, 155–69

pharmacies, 77
physical health, community care and, 74
placement, versus integration, 72
Plessy v. Ferguson, 156
podcasts, 31–32
police encounters: avoiding, 7; crisis response teams and, 10–11, 48; disrespect and, 16; Marshall and, 4; neighborhood and, 6; personal experience of, 8–9, 12–16; Ramirez and, 180; Robbins and, 35–36; and violence, 12–17
policy: factors affecting, 191; peer participation in, 144–49
politics: disclosure of mental illness and, 139–40; voting patterns and, 152–53
post-traumatic stress disorder (PTSD), 24
poverty: and homelessness, 85; and violence, 5
pretrial detention, 36–39
Princeton University, 122
prison: conditions in, 45–47; term, 34. *See also* jail
privacy: advocacy for, 138; and involuntary medication, 132
private health insurance, Smith and, 99
product test, 44
Project LETS, 123–25
providers: and possibility, 75–76; and stigma, 166–67
Providing Empathetic and Effective Recovery Support Act (PEER Support Act), 114–15, 148, 194

psychiatric advance directives, 146, 206
psychiatric survivors, term, 125, 172
punishment, justifications for, 42–43

quality of life: ACT model and, 57; Fountain House and, 70
questions, open-ended, 64

race: and mental illness, 5, 156–58, 177–78; and police encounters, 13
racism, and homelessness, 85
RAISE-ETP, 119–20
Ramirez, Hector, 170–71, 180–81
REACT, 88, 90–91, 93–95
Reagan, Ronald, 54
recovery: Fountain House and, 70; goal of, 78; nature of, ix, 197–98; Smith and, 64; term, viii; timeframe of, 176
recovery models, x, 192c, 192–93
red flag laws, 32–33
reentry services, 51–52
refusal of treatment, 173–74; hospitals and, 18; legal issues and, 59–63; personal experience of, 198–99
rehabilitation, 42
Rehabilitation Act, 195
religion: and mental illness, 177, 180; Smith and, 98–99
rent, The Other Side Village and, 92
residents, psychiatric, 75–76
respect, emergency departments and, 22
restoration services, 38–39
restraint: emergency departments and, 21; personal experience of, 202–6

retribution, 42–43
Richards, Mark, 57–58
rights: competency and, 38, 40; to liberty, 26; to refuse treatment, 59–63, 132; Second Amendment, 32, 134–36; to treatment, 19–20, 54–55
Risperdal, 75
Rivers, Lynn, 139
Robbins, Alaina Jean Marie, 35–36
Roberts, Marilyn, 166
Robinson principle, 42
Robinson v. California, 39–40, 86
Rodriguez, Rafael, 80–83, 93–96, 113
Rowling, J. K., 164
rural areas, crisis response in, 11

Saks, Elyn, 165
Salvation Army, 71
scattered site model, 93–95
schizophrenia: and combating self-stigma, 184; fear of, 186–87; gender and, 178; RAISE-ETP and, 119; and violence, 5, 59, 162
Schur, Lisa, 152
Scopelitis family, 142
seclusion: emergency departments and, 21; personal experience of, 200–201, 204
self-actualization, 193
self-advocacy, 188
self-esteem: education and, 117; employment and, 183–84; Fountain House and, 70
self-harm, solitary confinement and, 37
self-help groups, 181–85

self-stigma, 171, 188; combating, 181–85
serious mental illness (SMI): employment and, 102; and homelessness, 79; jail and, 34–35; term, vii
service user, term, 171
sexual violence: Frost and, 178; Rodriguez and, 80
Shadur, Milton, 111
Shaw-Rosenbaum, Rachael, 121
shelters, peer-run, 87
Shelton, Richard, 76
shortages: hospital beds, 20, 85; housing, 87; staff, 56, 74, 194
Simone, Nina, 164
Slack, Joel, 146
Smith, Eric, 63–66, 118
Smith, Ivanova, 149
Smith, Samantha, 98–101, 145, 177
soccer, 183
social distance, and stigma, 161
social media, and advocacy, 145
solitary confinement, 37
Soteria-Alaska, 131, 136–37
Sotomayor, Sonia, 87
staffing ratios: Bryce Hospital and, 19; minimum requirements for, 20
staffing shortages, 74, 194; and community treatment options, 56
staircase metaphor, 53–54, 78
stand-alone psychiatric emergency programs, 23
Stefan, Susan, 122
Steinl, Kevin, 21
stigma, 159–62, 190–91; combating, 163–67; disclosure and, 112; and education, 116; Fountain House and, 70; internalized, 171, 181–85, 188; peer support and, 57; Project LETS and, 125; race and, 177; term, 159–60; terminology and, 171–74; and trans identity, 179
Sting, 175
Street Crisis Response Team (SCRT), 47–48
stress: hiding diagnosis and, 140; lawyers and, 133
students, and peer support, 121–26
Substance Abuse and Mental Health Services Administration (SAMHSA), 147–49
substance use disorder: and housing issues, 94; and violence, 5
success: factors affecting, x; REACT model and, 90
suicide: college and, 121–22, 124–25; guns and, 134; involuntary hospitalization and, 27; jail and, 37, 46
supervision, and peer support, 114
Supported Education, 120–21
Supported Employment, 104–5
supported housing, 90
support groups, personal experience of, 77–78
Supreme Court, 86–87; *Dred Scott v. Sandford*, 156; *Kahler v. Kansas*, 41–42

Taney, Roger B., 156
Tasers, 12
Teresa, mother, 174
terminology, x–xi, 171–74
Texas, 100
Thompson, Myron, 147

tiny home communities, 95
training: and employment, 104–5; for helpline, 126; for mentors, 123
trans identity, and mental illness, 178–80
transitional employment, 108
trauma: peer crisis response and, 10; personal experience of, 200–201
travel, and self-confidence, 183
treatment: involuntary, 18; involuntary hospitalization and, 19–20; jails and, 45–47; rights to, 19–20
Trump, Donald, 114, 147–48, 152–53, 194
trust: ACT model and, 58; failure of, personal experience of, 203–4; lived experience and, 82
Turner, Ted, 164

unemployment: and homelessness, 85; and people with mental illness, 102–4
United States v. Brawner, 44
Utah, 91–93

Van Dyke, Jason, 13
Vars, Caroline, ix, 8, 13, 75, 198, 205
victim mentality, 172
violence: factors affecting, 5; and fear, 162–63; homeless individuals and, 85; police encounters and, 12–17; statistics on, 4–5
Virginia, 144
visitor policies, 199–200, 205
voices, hearing, 186–87; education on, 166–67; Myers and, 131; Pagdon and, 116–17

Volpe, Justin, 168
Voluntary Do-Not-Sell Firearms List, 134–36, 141–44
voluntary hospitalization, 55
voting, 152–53

Wade, Morgan, 176
waiting periods, and gun purchases, 135–36
Wallace, Jamie Lee, 45–47
Wallace, Mike, 164
Wang, Luchang, 121
Washington, 143, 149
weapons: and dangerousness, 12; gun laws and, 134–36, 141–44, 149–51; red flag laws and, 32–33
Weicker, Lowell, 145
West, Kanye, 175
Wettengel, Melissa, 73–74, 113–14
Whitaker, Bob, 131
Wildflower Alliance, 81, 93, 113
Wilson, Diane, 54–55
Wood, Annette, 152
work as peer support: challenges of, 113–14; and expectations, 154; and identity, 182; lived experience and, 53; and recovery, 73, 77–78
Wyatt, Ricky, 24–25
Wyatt standards, 20
Wyatt v. Stickney, 19–20, 54, 105

Yale University, 121–23
Young, Amanda Adcock, 134

Zeller, Scott, 22
Zeta-Jones, Catherine, 164

www.ingramcontent.com/pod-product-compliance
Ingram Content Group UK Ltd.
Pitfield, Milton Keynes, MK11 3LW, UK
UKHW041036150426
5221IPUK00008B/29